Peppermint

About the author
Jennifer Britt is a journalist and writer with a special interest in health and natural medicine. She has co-authored a
book on the medicinal herb, feverfew.

Peppermint

A traditional herbal remedy and modern plant medicine

Jennifer Britt

Silver Link Publishing Ltd

First published in 1992

British Library Cataloguing in Publication Data

A catalogue record for this book is available from the British Library.

ISBN 0 947971 97 1

Silver Link Publishing Ltd
Unit 5
Home Farm Close
Church Street
Wadenhoe
Peterborough PE8 5TE

Printed and bound in Great Britain by
Cox & Wyman Ltd, Reading, Berkshire

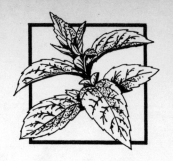

Contents

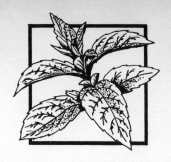

Acknowledgements

I am grateful for all the help I have received in writing this book; to Dr Brian Evans, for his advice and the loan of his PhD thesis; and to Dr Douglas Holdstock and medical herbalist Rosalind Blackwell who shared their expertise generously and read large chunks of the manuscript. If any errors have slipped into the final version, it is entirely due to me, not to them.

Thanks are also due to others, especially: Mark Bennett of Bennett Natural Products; Judith Smallwood of Judith Smallwood Public Relations; Timothy Whittaker of Potter's (Herbal Supplies) Ltd; Vic Perfitt of Gerard House Ltd; staff at Power Health Products Ltd; Russell McGuinness of Wilson & Mansfield Ltd; Larry Glick of Tillomed Laboratories Ltd; medical herbalist Carol Church; aromatherapist Katrina Roberts; Dr Stan Deans of the Scottish Agricultural College; Rosemary Titterington of Iden Croft Herbs; Judith Hopkinson of Hollington Nurseries; Mrs Joy Mason, Lone Dantoff; and Ann Warren-Davis of the Herb Society. Above all I am grateful to my husband Robert, for his support and patience, and likewise to my son Christopher, who says my next book ought to be for him.

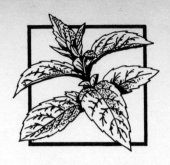

Foreword

by Jan de Vries

It is with the greatest pleasure that I write the foreword for this most useful and interesting book about peppermint. A traditional remedy with a long history of use, peppermint is also an important medicine for today, especially as the findings from modern medical and scientific research mean that more than ever before is understood about the medicinal properties of this plant.

Today's wide use of peppermint as a herbal food supplement is due in no small measure to the work of Erhardt Obbekjaer during the 1970s. His enthusiasm generated a new popular interest in the use of oil of peppermint in his native Denmark, and then further afield as products bearing his name became widely available in Europe.

My own experience of using peppermint during more than three decades in natural health practice is that it is an excellent natural remedy. Over the years I have used it successfully in the treatment of thousands of patients without any side effects. I have found peppermint to be a real friend in practice, being particularly helpful in conditions such as irritable bowel syndrome, and those resulting from microbial activity. In its various forms peppermint is also recommended for treating indigestion, nausea, diarrhoea, colds, headaches, flatulence, and cramps.

I would like to congratulate the author of this informative, helpful and easy-to-read book, who shares her knowledge most interestingly, and I wish all the readers of *Peppermint* good health.

Jan de Vries

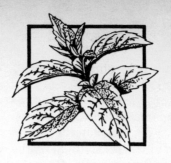

Introduction

Peppermint is one of the most commonplace of herbal extracts in modern British households, widely used in toilet preparations and confectionery. For many people, as they pick up the toothpaste, peppermint may be the first thing they taste in the morning, and the final breath-freshening flavour of the evening.

But for all its domestic familiarity, peppermint is no longer so much associated with the family medicine cupboard, where it would have often been found a couple of generations ago. Yet this is arguably its most valuable role.

Peppermint is not an "olde worlde remedie" that has been surpassed by modern alternatives, but a medicinal substance which has stood the test of time.

The plant we now know as peppermint (*Mentha piperita*) was distinguished as a species of mint 300 years ago and has had a clear record of medicinal use since then. It is part of an even older tradition of "mint medicine" because other species of mint have a history, going back thousands of years, as remedies for conditions in which peppermint is still found to be effective.

Modern scientific research is confirming the validity of many of peppermint's traditional uses and today this plant extract is not only prescribed by specialists in herbal medicine, but is also available on the National Health Service for treating the common condition, irritable bowel syndrome.

And as a first aid remedy in the home, it does safe, sterling service, with its low risk of side effects and its broad range of applications - in digestive upsets, colds and catarrh, headaches, for skin conditions and pain relief.

Dried peppermint can simply be made into a tea, but the most usual method of concentrating the plant's medicinal properties is to extract its oil to make into capsules and tablets and other convenient forms.

This book offers a guide to its medicinal uses, as well as describing its cultivation and tracing some of the history behind peppermint, the modern plant medicine.

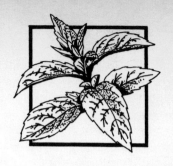

CHAPTER ONE

Mint in history

History books and old herbals give tantalising hints that *Mentha piperita*, the plant we popularly know as peppermint, was familiar to people as diverse as the ancient Assyrians, Egyptians and medieval Icelanders.

But it was much later in history and closer to home that the plant, which is today one of the world's most abundantly-produced and economically important medicinal herbs, was recorded for posterity as a distinct type of mint . . . in Home Counties England by a 17th-century Essex man.

John Ray (1627-1705), who usually gets the credit for coining the name "peper mint", was a lad of humble origins who made good, the son of a blacksmith at Black Notley, a village near Braintree. His mother was the community's "wise" woman who prepared herbal remedies from local plants for sick villagers. Ray (originally his name was Wray) was possessed of a boundless curiosity for all aspects of the natural world and had exceptional intellectual gifts. Described as the most distinguished British naturalist of the 17th century, his was a spectacular academic career. At 16, having been encouraged from an early age by the then vicar of Braintree, Samuel Collins, he won a scholarship to Cambridge University and, on gaining his degree, lectured in Hebrew, Greek, Latin, Mathematics and the Humanities.

A period of enforced leisure, following an illness, gave him the opportunity to roam Cambridgeshire, testing his theory that plant life varied from place to place. It was the start of his systematic exploration of local floras throughout Britain, in Europe and further afield.

Ray recorded peppermint as a distinct species of the mint genus in his 1696 *Synopsis of British Plants*, one of many works he published on a wide range of subjects. He described it in exaggerated terms, as a mint with a "fiery taste of pepper" (sapore fervido piperis). In 1704, in his *Historia Plantarum*, Ray named the plant as *Mentha palustris*, the name *Mentha piperita* coming later from the pen of the Swedish botanist Linnaeus*. Soon "peper mint" was found to be a particularly medicinally-useful mint (due to its high menthol content).

It was not long before peppermint was being classified by many botanists as a cross breed between spearmint and water mint. For all that it was an Englishman of the 1600s who put the peppermint species on the modern botanical map of the world, it is probable that types of mint very similar to it had been growing for hundreds, perhaps thousands of years, if not in England, then in other countries and under different names.

There are possible associations with some of the oldest civilisations. Assyrian herbal texts refer to green urnu, taken to be peppermint, as opposed to urnu, which was probably garden mint, spearmint[1]. Mrs Mary (Maud) Grieve, a herb grower, fellow of the Royal Horticultural Society and the author behind a formidably comprehen-

---

* Some botanists have disputed whether the plant that Linnaeus identified as *Mentha piperita* was the same as Ray's "peper mint", but that's another story.

sive tome, *A Modern Herbal*, originally published in 1931*, says that there is evidence that *Mentha piperita* was cultivated by the Egyptians, much of whose medicinal knowledge was inherited by the later ancient Grecian civilisation.

Some scholars believe that the Greek-born physician to the Roman army, Pedanius Dioscorides (1st century AD) may be referring to peppermint, or something very similar, when he describes in his *De Materia Medica* (a source of information about healing plants of the day and the basis of many subsequent medieval herbals) a form of mint with warming, contractive power[2]. According to Mrs Grieve, peppermint was also mentioned in a 13th-century Icelandic pharmacopoeia, although she does not elaborate.

When it comes to mint in general, there is written evidence of its use in ancient societies, in ways similar to those of peppermint in modern times, going back over several millennia.

An early written record of mint as a medicine comes from Babylon of the era of King Hammurabi (circa 2000 BC), who devised a pre-Hippocratic code of medical practice[3]; stone tablets from the public records office refer to many plants noted for their curative value. Among them was *Mentha viridis*, or spearmint as we commonly call it[4].

The traditional Chinese pharmacopoeia, the Pen Ts'ao (or Ben Cao) refers to several mints[5], but it is not clear how ancient their inclusion is. Folklore traces the knowledge originally recorded in the Pen Ts'ao to the herbalist-Emperor Shen Nung (or Shen Nong) a part-legendary, part-historic figure, whose life is linked to various dates, the earliest being around 3,494 BC[6]. Even once it was in

---

* It was based on Mrs Grieve's pamphlets and edited by Mrs Hilda Leyel, founder of the Society of Herbalists[4].

written form, this herbal encylopaedia appeared in a
number of expanding versions over the centuries, culmi-
nating in the still-influential work of physician and phar-
macologist Dr Li Shih Ch'en[7] who lived 400 years ago.

Mint was used widely in ancient Greece and became
immortalised in Greek mythology with the story (or one
version of it) of how Persephone, the jealous queen of
Pluto, King of the Underworld, on learning of his adul-
tery with the beautiful nymph, Minthe, crushed her.
Although Pluto did not have the power to bring his
beloved back fully restored, he did give her new life as a
plant.

From a 20th century perspective, there is an aura of the
exotic and mysterious about anything associated with
people who lived thousands of years ago, but in the
households of antiquity, mint was probably just as much
an everyday practical domestic herb as it is for us. Mint
remedies must have soothed many a troubled ancient
Greek, and later Roman, tum. It was used in dental preparations, as a soothing infusion for haemorrhoids[1] and an
air freshener. The Athenian comic poet Antiphanes (4th
century BC) describes the elaborate toilet of the rich
Greek:

"He bathes
In a large gilded tub, and steeps his feet
And legs in rich Egyptian unguent:
His jaws and breasts he rubs with thick palm oil
And both his arms with extract sweet, of *mint*; . . ."[8]

A rich source of information about how ancient peoples
used plants is the Bible. It is in the New Testament, in the
gospels of Luke and Matthew, that we find references to
mint - two versions of a saying, attributed to Jesus, about
the paying of tithes by Pharisees, the grass-roots religious
teachers of the time (the common Christian perception of

them as narrow-minded subscribers to the letter, rather than the spirit, of Jewish law is today challenged by a number of biblical scholars). Though learned, they were also working people and many of them must have worked the land . . . contributing a tenth of what they produced. Luke quotes Jesus: "But woe unto you, Pharisees, for ye tithe mint and rue and all manner of herbs and pass over judgement and the love of God." (Luke 11,42).

The moral usually extracted from these words is that people can become so obsessed with the minutiae of religious duty - like tithing tiny quantities of domestic herbs such as mint - that more profound spirituality passes them by. The glimpse we can extract from the story into the life of Palestine 2,000 years ago is of an agricultural society. As well as field crops, herbs and vegetables were grown on small kitchen garden plots near the houses.

As a seasoning, mint seems to have been used in many foods in the kitchens of former civilisations. The gourmet Marcus Apicius, who flourished in the Roman heyday years of the 1st century AD, used it frequently in his recipes.

The Roman Pliny the Elder, writing his vast encyclopaedic *Natural History* in the same era says that mint ". . . is agreeable for stuffing cushions and pervades the tables with its scent at country banquets". "It refreshes our spirits and its flavour gives a zest to food". "By itself mint prevents milk from turning sour or curdled and thick."[9]

During Pliny's lifetime the Romans invaded Celtic Britain (AD 43) and as mint was probably originally a native plant of the Mediterranean and Middle and Far East, one theory is that the occupying forces, who carried all kinds of seeds and plants to the outposts of their vast empire[4], brought it across the English Channel.

There was also an ancient native healing inheritance which pre-dated the Romans and survived the years of periodic upheaval following their withdrawal from

Britain and the waves of invading Angles and Saxons. The emerging Anglo-Saxon medical practice combined native Celtic knowledge with Germanic pagan herbal lore and classical traditions all within the framework of the new Christian philosophy.

Religious houses became centres of medical information and practical doctoring. Medieval monasteries and abbeys had their own herb gardens, a fine example of which has been recreated at Shaftesbury Abbey in Dorset, a Benedictine foundation of King Alfred (of burnt-cakes fame) whose daughter Aelfgyfa became the first abbess in 888[10].

Later famed for its miracles associated with the tomb of a Saxon martyred king, St Edward, Shaftesbury became an important healing centre, and the nuns grew many medicinal plants. The herb garden there today includes two mints, pennyroyal (*Mentha pulegium*) and water mint (*Mentha aquatica*).

There is a similar venture at the excavated Benedictine monastery of Jarrow, now incorporated into the Bede Monastery Museum in Tyne & Wear. A surviving plan of a physician's garden drawn up in 9th-century Switzerland at St Gall, used as reference in Jarrow, includes mint and pennyroyal[11].

Initially it was the training provided by the religious houses that helped foster a new breed of professional physicians. There was also folk medicine practised and passed on through the ages by lay people (the "wise men and women"). Knowledge was inherited particularly from mother to daughter, and even today there are echoes of personal reminiscence of this tradition. A few years ago a local historian in Surrey was presented with a still, used by several generations of one village family for distilling oil from peppermint and other plants to supply to the local doctors. This practice had continued until the First World War era. The woman who made the gift had not carried on her family's tradition, but her mother, grand-mother and great grandmother had all served the village as herbal distillers.

As well as the specialists, most women in past centuries acquired knowledge of plants for various domestic uses.

Tudor physician William Turner in his *Herball* tells us that the garden mint in the mid-1500s was "spere mynte"[12] and master-surgeon John Gerard, writing a few years later in his *Great Herball or General Historie of Plantes*, says: "The savor or smell of the Water Mint rejoyceth the heart of man for which cause they use to strew it in chambers and places of recreation, pleasure and repose, where feasts and banquets are made."[13]

The apothecary Nicholas Culpeper, in the following century, informs us that a mint gargle cures sore mouths and gums and "ill-savoured breath" and is useful for washing children's heads when they are inclined to sores."[14]

Even in the late 19th century, when new pharmaceutical medicines were starting to edge out traditional herbal remedies, Flora Thompson in *Lark Rise*, the first book of her 'Lark Rise to Candleford' trilogy, which records a time-honoured way of country life then already on its way to extinction, describes how poor but self-sufficient village women grew herbs in their cottage gardens. Thyme, parsley and sage for the cooking pot, rosemary to flavour the home-made lard, lavender to scent the best clothes, and horehound, camomile, tansy, balm, rue, pen-nyroyal and peppermint as medicine. Peppermint tea was drunk, not so much medicinally, but as a luxury: "It was brought out on special occasions and drunk from wine glasses."[15]

For townies unable to grow their own, mint was a basic item in the apothecary's shop, the forerunner of our mod-ern pharmacies. A Dr Westmacott, writing in 1694 about such establishments, which also provided affordable, basic medical advice for the poorer classes unable to afford a physician, describes the forms of mint they supplied: "1. The Dry Herbs. 2ndly. Mint Water. 3rdly. Spirit of Mints. 4th. Syrup of Mints. 5th. The Conserve of Leaves. 6th. The Simple Oyl. 7th The Chemical Oyl."[12]

The *London Pharmacopoeia* specifically listed peppermint for the first time in 1721, and Mitcham in Surrey became well-known from the late 1700s onwards as the source of abundant quantities of peppermint and other herbs for druggists and apothecaries in the fast-growing capital, a 9-mile cart-ride away. Towards the end of the 18th century there were 250 acres given over to physic gardens, with peppermint being by far the biggest crop. Just a few years later one of the leading growers was a James Moore (of Potter & Moore fame) who in Victorian Mitcham farmed 543 acres, producing mainly peppermint.[16]

Famed also for its lavender, this peppermint-growing and distilling area spread as far as Kingston, Croydon and Chipstead. Because the lavender and peppermint harvests usually fell during the same period, extra hands would be drafted in, with whole families coming over from Ireland to help before moving on to Kent for the hop picking, according to a 1901 report in *Country Life* magazine.[16]

Growing continued in the 20th century, but the heyday of Mitcham peppermint was past; production in the US and elsewhere was already making an impact.

In Mary Grieve's day, Mitcham peppermint and other English crops of the herb were considered "incomparably" superior to others. The problem, however, was that the wet, cloudy English climate produced quality but not quantity of oil, making it more expensive and uncompetitive. Some mints are still grown in Britain today, but not peppermint on a large, commercial scale.

Mrs Grieve[12] speculates that the Pilgrim Fathers first planted mint in America, but opinions vary about when peppermint was first cultivated there. Certainly it was being grown by the early 1800s, and the United States later became the world's foremost producer.

By the start of this century, Japanese mint or peppermint (*Mentha arvensis*), which was useful because of its high content of menthol, was already an important herb crop in Japan, where it supplied a flourishing oil-distilling and menthol-extracting industry. (China and Brazil are now much bigger producers of *Mentha arvensis*.) Mrs Grieve relates how the Japanese had long recognised the benefits of menthol and had traditionally carried it about with them "in little silver boxes hanging from their girdles".

Rather more prosaically, referring to pre-1930s Britain, she writes about sanitary engineers using peppermint oil to test the tightness of pipe joints, because its pungent odour identified any leaks, and of rat-catchers soaking rags in the stuff to drive rats, who had an aversion to the aroma, from their holes. That now sounds delightfully quaint, but the same section also has references to peppermint's medicinal uses as an antispasmodic, an anaesthetic and an antiseptic which remain as current today as they were when Mrs Grieve was writing . . . and as they had been for many centuries before.

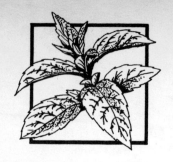

CHAPTER TWO

Mint, a traditional medicine

Indigestion, tummy pain, bowel troubles, a blocked up nose, a headache: a modern-day herbal might well recommend peppermint as suitable treatment for any of these conditions. Pliny, the 1st-century AD Roman scholar, gave similar advice. He was not familiar with the name peppermint, but he was well-versed in the properties of mint in general.

". . . a three-fingered pinch of the dried powder taken in water relieves stomach ache . . .," he writes in his *Natural History*, which summarises the knowledge of natural science of his day. "It stays . . . violent disturbance of the bowels, if taken in water with starch . . ." "It is applied . . . to rectal troubles . . ." "With pomegranate juice . . . it stops hiccough and vomiting." "It is also applied to the temples for headache." "The juice of fresh mint inhaled is good for affections of the nostrils."[9]

The work of Pliny and other contemporary scholars and writers such as the Greco-Roman physician Dioscorides was shaped by knowledge that had been handed on to them from previous generations. Their writing in turn continued to influence medical thought for many centuries afterwards. The illustrated guide to medicinal plants, the *Materia Medica* of Dioscorides, was the basis for many medieval and even later herbals. Words originally formed by the quills of antiquity are repeated down the ages.

When London apothecary and botanist John Parkinson wrote his comprehensive guide to drugs of the day, the *Theatre of Plants*, in 1640, he was not only expounding the then current practice, but also summarising the still-influential opinions on medicinal plants of experts from hundreds, even thousands, of years ago. Parkinson was writing in the great age of herbals, when, thanks to the invention of the printing press, such works appeared in greater than ever numbers.

Yet in discussing the alleged aphrodisiac properties of mint, he still refers to the Greek Aristotle who had lived around 1,800 years before: "Aristotle and others in ancient times forbade mints to be used of souldiers in the time of warre because they thought it did much to incite venery, that it took away or at least abated their animosity of courage to fight."[17]

There is, however, a divergence of opinion in Parkinson's pages about mint's effect on sexual appetites, because he also says that one of the virtues of wild mints is that they "helpe the pollutions in the night, used both inwardly and the juyce being applied outwardly to the testicles and cod." *

Mint had other applications in matters reproductive, according to Parkinson: "Applyed to the privie parts of women before the act of generation it hindreth conception." *

He recommends it for repressing milk in swollen breasts, also for "such as have swollen, flagging or great breasts" and, more reminiscent of current practice in which peppermint does have applications in treating menstrual disorders: "It is of especiall use to stay the femi-

*Neither use is to be recommended!

nine courses when they come on too fast."

Mint's effectiveness in relieving the biting of a "mad dogge" and against the poison of "venemous creatures" might not justify its inclusion in today's family medicine cupboard, but many of Parkinson's recommendations remain relevant.

". . . it is very profitable to the stomach." "The vertues of the wild mints are more especially to dissolve winde in the stomache."

It is good for the head and memory, he says: "Not onely to be smelled unto, but chiefly to be applyed unto the head and temples and easeth the headache."

". . . the decoction or distilled water helpeth a stinking breath, which proceedeth from corruption of the teeth and snuffed up into the nose purgeth the head."

Once peppermint had been distinguished as a species, some 30 years after Parkinson was writing, it became the most popular medicinal mint and was described in the early 1700s as superior to other mints for stomach complaints and diarrhoea.

An important step towards a modern scientific understanding of peppermint's pharmacological properties was the isolating of menthol by German scientists in 1771[2], although the word menthol came later.

The peppermint species was soon being grown abroad, often being referred to as English mint (Menthe Anglaise in French, for example) and in 1797 a pharmaceutical chemist from Erfurt in Germany, Johann Trommsdorf[2], had opened a factory extracting ethereal oils from peppermint and other plants.

There are numerous references to the use of peppermint in records of popular medicine from around the world.

A Danish pharmacopoeia of 1772 describes it as one of the most widely-used household remedies[2]. In Denmark, too, frostbitten hands were treated with peppermint, and the plant extract, along with camomile flowers, was put in hot footbaths, and used for treating eczema[2].

In Germany a wine extract of peppermint and curled mint, camomile flowers and black breadcrumbs was used as a compress for children's dysentery, and a domestic Russian remedy for ulcers was a tea of peppermint, gentian, sage and cinnamon[2].

In Latvia it was recommended for whooping cough, in the Ukraine peppermint leaves, lilac and balsam, olive oil and unsalted butter were tied on malignant boils[2].

The references are legion and the uses immensely varied, but consistent is peppermint's applications in digestive problems, fevers, colds and headaches.

Although neither peppermint nor other kinds of mint were believed to be native to the American continent, European settlers had introduced it by the end of the 18th century. Samuel Stearn in *The American Herbal* of 1801 notes that it was being grown in gardens. "It is a stimulant," he says. "It restores the functions of the stomach, promotes digestion, stops vomiting, cures the hiccups, flatulent colic, hysterical depressions and other like complaints. It does not heat the constitution so much as might be expected."[18]

Native Americans, with their own fine inheritance of botanical medicine, also started using peppermint. A major survey of the ethnic uses of plants, carried out in the 1920s among the already badly decimated native populations, included the medicines of the 1,745 remaining members of the Menomini tribe, then living on a reservation in Shawano country in north-eastern Wisconsin. They called peppermint "cold water, as it tastes", and they used it as one ingredient in a tea or poultice for pneumonia.[19]

Peppermint's classic association with relief of flatulence was the cause of some laboured humour on the part of an English doctor, Dr W. T. Fernie, a prolific writer of popular medical books with a penchant for the poetic and for classical allusions. From his *Meals Medicinal* (1905)[20]:

"Anise and mint with strong Aeolian sway,
Intestinal storms of flatulence allay."

Dr Fernie also refers to peppermint's use in tuberculosis: "As an antiseptic and destroyer of germs, this oil is remarkably efficacious, on which account it is advised for inhalation by consumptive patients."[20]

Writing some years later, Alfred Hall, a fellow of the National Institute of Medical Herbalists and a member of the Pharmaceutical Society, confirms that oils of peppermint and of eucalyptus are "excellent to use in pulmonary tuberculosis."[21]

He also says that the oil acts as an anaesthetic and "painted along the course of an inflamed nerve it will often give long relief until more permanent methods can be used."

He used it in herpes and shingles, combined it with capsicum and oil of wintergreen as a topical application in rheumatism and sciatica, and in a wash for ulcerated mouths for gum disease and after the extraction of teeth.

"It relieves gastric and intestinal colic and flatulence and if taken in hot water, the relief is almost instantaneous," he says.

Today medical herbalists comprise a small specialist branch of medicine, a reflection of the way in which during the last 100 years plant medicines in the developed world have increasingly been supplanted by pharmaceutical drugs.

Yet the 20th century has also seen another steady development; the scientific analysis of the pharmacological properties of plant extracts, the results of which have helped foster the current revival of serious interest in the medicinal value of plant material. Experiments with the volatile oils of various plants from the early 1900s onwards have in particular helped illuminate some aspects of peppermint's pharmacology.

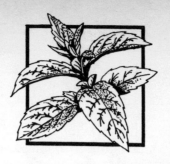

CHAPTER THREE

Peppermint explained

In many societies in the past, understanding and practice of medicine were bound up with magical or religious beliefs. The action of plants on the body was often attributed to supernatural influence rather than to their own natural properties. Even today herbal medicines are sometimes popularly described in terms such as magic potions, wonder remedies and the like. But to use such descriptions does plant medicines a disservice because it makes it easier to relegate them to the fringe.

The effects of plant medicines, far from defying the modern scientific understanding of how human bodies and drugs interact, are explained more fully by it. It may seem miraculous that everything that exists is fashioned from numerous different combinations of just 92 naturally-occurring chemical elements (approximately 24 make up the human body), and that the whole cycle of life boils down to a systematic chain of chemical reactions. It is also the most basic fact of science and it means that plant medicines like peppermint are no more or less magical than synthetic drugs. They are all composed of chemicals which, when they interact with the human chemical system, cause a change which should (as long as the medical diagnosis and the choice of medicine are correct) help the body to function more efficiently.

In the case of peppermint, not everything there is to be known about its chemical constituents and the effects they have on the human system has yet been analysed and documented. There is much about the healing properties of peppermint which is not fully understood, but this is not because it is beyond the wit of scientists to get to grips with every aspect of the plant's chemistry, but because like many plants it is chemically complex, and to study it exhaustively would entail a vast amount of work. There is, after all, a huge choice of research projects offered by the plant kingdom alone, let alone the rest of the natural world, and only so many scientists, so much time and so much money to go round.

During the 1980s the growing realisation among doctors and in the pharmaceutical industry that peppermint, particularly its extracted oil, is extremely useful as a medicine provided an added impetus to research. As a result, some aspects of its chemistry and the intricacies of how this affects the human body, particularly in irritable bowel syndrome for which peppermint has become a routinely prescribed treatment, have been investigated in new depth.

But oil of peppermint is a combination of many chemicals and groups of chemicals and it is mainly the pharmacology of its menthol content that has been studied. Moreover, much of the research has been on extracted menthol, rather than on whole peppermint, the form in which it is used in herbal and often in allopathic medicine.

Specialists in herbal medicines also use it as a treatment in many conditions which have so far not attracted the attention of conventional scientific researchers. A comprehensive survey of the medicinal properties attributed to peppermint still has to refer a great deal to the accumulated evidence from practitioners observing the effects it produces when administered to patients.

Many practitioners and pharmacologists might say that though they know that peppermint seems to work in various medicinal ways, they do not know exactly how and why. Their knowledge of human physiology and plant chemistry nevertheless enables them to make educated guesses.

What it contains

Peppermint is a combination of many chemical compounds: esters, aldehydes, alcohols, ketones and terpenes. The volatile oils of peppermint are the source of most of its medicinal properties, with menthol being the key active ingredient, but the other constituents may also contribute to the plant's therapeutic effects.

Menthol is a monoterpene, it can also be described as an alcohol, and forms, according to various estimates, between 30% and 70% of peppermint *oil*[22]. In an extract of the whole plant that proportion is lower, whereas in Japanese peppermint oil it is higher, between around 64% and 89%[23].

Peppermint and the digestive system

Peppermint has a well-proven antispasmodic - relaxing - effect on smooth muscle, the type of muscle of which the walls of the intestines and the stomach, and also blood vessels, are made. The antispasmodic action of peppermint on the intestines has been studied in laboratory and clinical studies more extensively than any of its other properties, mainly in relation to its application in irritable bowel syndrome (see Chapters 4 and 5).

Smooth muscle, so-called because of its tissue texture, is also known as involuntary muscle, in that its movements are not under our conscious control as are those of

a skeletal muscle. Skeletal muscle attached to our bones
goes into action, helping to bend an arm for instance,
when we consciously decide that is what we want to do.
The movement of the intestines is partly intrinsic, but
modified by the part of the brain which is on "automatic
pilot".

Movement of muscle, triggered by nerve impulses from
the brain, is basically contraction followed by relaxation.
It is this rhythmic motion that enables the smooth muscle
of the stomach and intestines to carry out its function of
propelling food through the digestive tract.

The intestines do not contract and relax continuously;
they do so when there is food to digest and evacuate, and
their movement is triggered by messages, stimuli like
electric impulses, sent from elsewhere in the gut and from
the brain. These neurotransmitters change the voltage in
the muscle wall cells, which are all like tiny batteries, so
that they momentarily change shape. Basically they
squash up - contract - and the muscle becomes shortened
and thickened. They then spring back into shape and the
muscle is stretchy and relaxed again until, ping, another
neurotransmitter hits the muscle wall and the process
restarts.

The chemistry behind contractions is that each neurotransmitter alters the balance between sodium and potas-
sium within and outside the cells, which allows in a tiny
amount of additional calcium. This is quite normal and
presents no problem until some hiccup in the system
makes the intestines contract faster or more violently, and
therefore more painfully, than usual; the desired effect
then is to make the muscles more relaxed. The menthol in
peppermint is believed to block off the channels by which
the calcium comes into the cells, reducing the intensity -
and pain - of the contractions.

The term *carminative* is an overall way of describing
remedies that have a soothing effect on the digestive sys-

tem, easing flatulence (wind) and colic. Peppermint is a carminative partly because of its antispasmodic properties, but there may be at least one other mode of action here.

The effectiveness of peppermint in expelling wind - either air trapped in the digestive tract or gas produced by the breakdown of foods in the stomach - has long been observed and can be explained partly by its ability to relax the intestines. A test-tube experiment[24] also suggested that peppermint helps break down gastric and intestinal foams in which gas can become trapped in the small intestine, so aiding its passage out of the system.

Peppermint can also relieve wind and gas in the stomach, helping to bring it up, rather than down, by relaxing the muscle (oesophageal sphincter) that controls the opening between the stomach and the oesophagus (the muscular tube connecting the stomach and the throat, known colloquially as the gullet). This action on the oesophageal sphincter can also cause the unwelcome regurgitation of acid with resulting irritation of the gullet, heartburn.[25]

Peppermint also has other actions in the stomach - sometimes it is referred to as a *stomachic*; in particular it has a mild anaesthetic effect on the stomach wall which alleviates nausea and quells the desire to vomit.

Peppermint and the liver

Like many plant medicines, peppermint is a *hepatic*, with a broad-ranging effect on the liver. Herbal medicine puts a great deal of emphasis on the healthy working of the liver, which is a large gland with multifarious tasks in aiding digestion, metabolism of nutrients and cleaning out of toxins, so under-par liver function is suspected to be a contributory factor in many seemingly unrelated conditions.

Peppermint influences one of the liver's key functions,

the supply of bile, which affects the healthy working of the bowel. Bile is a substance through which the liver excretes toxins which otherwise would be building up both in the liver and elsewhere around the body. Bile also breaks down fat so that the body can digest and absorb it.

The liver cells (the hepatic cells) secrete around a quart of bile every day, which makes its way to the intestines, either to be excreted or to help metabolise fat, through a network of capillaries and ducts. Bile which is not needed immediately in the intestine is stored in the gall bladder.

Peppermint has been observed to stimulate both the secretion of bile (an action described as *choleretic*) and its flow from the gall bladder (for which it is known as a *cholagogue*)[26] [27]. Menthol's effect on liver enzymes suggests that it has hormone-like properties, similar to progesterone[28].

Menthol and gallstones

A proprietary drug, containing menthol among other ingredients, has been shown to help dissolve gallstones[28] by inhibiting synthesis of cholesterol and fatty acids in the liver[26].

Peppermint as a peripheral vasodilator and diaphoretic

Peppermint is also noted as a peripheral vasodilator[27] having a relaxing or dilating action on the smooth muscle of the blood vessels, improving circulation and therefore proving useful in conditions like chilblains. It is not that blood vessels need to be perpetually fully dilated for healthy circulation . . . a certain degree of contraction or constriction is necessary. However, if they become too constricted and impede blood flow, dilation is then desirable. There are times when the body produces its own internal vasodilating substances - after exercise, for instance, when hard-worked muscles need an increased flow of blood carrying the oxygen needed to replace their depleted supplies. Peppermint and other plant substances with similar properties aid this action.

Peppermint's diaphoretic (sweat-inducing) effect is linked to its vasodilating properties because the stimulation of sweat glands can probably be partly attributed to the dilation of local blood vessels[27].

In herbal medicine a fever or temperature which accompanies an infectious illness, whether it is a cold, mild flu or a more serious condition, is regarded as part of the body's defence against infection. Medicines are selected to help the body cope with its fever rather than to suppress the temperature. Sweating is an important part of the process both because it is the body's own way of reducing temperature, and also because it helps to eliminate toxic wastes through the skin. In doing this it is acting as a back-up for the kidneys, which are the body's main detoxifying system.

In herbal practice peppermint is noted for both its cooling and heating properties when taken internally, its effect on temperature varying according to dose, circumstances and the condition of the patient[29]. The cooling effect is understood to be a consequence of peppermint's heating action. When peppermint is taken during a high temperature, the extra heat it produces in the body through increased circulation helps stimulate sweating which then brings the temperature down. Larger doses, especially if taken as a hot drink, and in a hot climate, increase peppermint's ultimate cooling effect. In lower temperatures peppermint will have a warming effect without encouraging perspiration, and there is no cooling as a result.

There is again this combination of cooling and heating properties when peppermint is applied to the skin to give local pain relief, but here a different rationale applies. Used topically, peppermint has an initial cooling effect, suggesting that the blood has been drawn away from the surface, which is then followed by a sensation of warmth. Because of this, peppermint has (rather confusingly considering its dilating action on blood vessels) also sometimes been said to have the opposite effect, that of making them contract or constrict. This is not as paradoxical as it first sounds. There are herbs which contain both chemicals that cause constriction and others which cause dilation. Researchers at the University of Siena in Italy[30] found that essential oil of rosemary worked like this. On being applied to the skin it would make the blood vessels near the surface constrict so that the blood was drawn away and the skin felt cool at first. But when the dilating effect of the oil started to work, the skin gradually warmed as the blood vessels relaxed and extra supplies of blood were brought to the area.

The researchers, however, detected only a small amount of the chemical compound pinene, which accounts for this mechanism, in peppermint.

The latest thinking and recent research presents an alternative explanation for peppermint's cool feel on the skin through its effect on the sensory nerve endings known as cold receptors, which keep the brain informed about the level of temperature in the outside environment, enabling it to adjust the body's own heating system. And as with the relaxing of smooth muscle, when you look at the basic biochemistry, peppermint, or more specifically menthol, appears to act on calcium channels. The cold receptors continually send reassuring messages back to the brain, informing it that the outside temperature requires no internal adjustments. Calcium seems to stimulate this negative feedback system[31], so when menthol interferes with its flow the brain immediately thinks the temperature outside has dropped and sends blood supplies speeding to the surface as protective warmth for the body. When peppermint is applied to the skin to relieve aches and pains, the initial coolness of its touch may alleviate the discomfort because of a slight numbing sensation, and then the increased blood flow will also help by cleansing and nourishing the area.

Peppermint in the respiratory tract

Peppermint has a reputation as an expectorant, a medicine which aids the removal of excess mucus from the lungs. Mucus in itself does not present a problem - it is a normal body fluid - but when it is secreted in excess, either in reaction to infection or an allergy, it makes it more difficult for the air to flow and causes congestion. Menthol in peppermint temporarily inhibits mucous secretion[32], hence its usefulness as an inhalant in conditions like asthma, bronchitis and colds.

Vapour from peppermint - either inhaled from steam or from a pill or lozenge sucked in the mouth - is often referred to as an anti-catarrhal or decongestant of nasal mucus. Recent research, however, indicates that peppermint does not reduce catarrh or make air flow more easily through the nose; instead it makes the body think that this is the effect it has had[33 34 35].

In one study 31 volunteers were administered with vapour of menthol and the level of resistance to air flow in their nasal passages was measured before and after with a special instrument, a nasal resistance meter, which involves breathing into a facemask[35]. There was no consistent increase in the rate of air flow, yet 22 of the volunteers said that they felt less congested. In fact, eight people who assured researchers that their noses felt much clearer, were found by the resistance meter to be more congested than before.

It is again the sensitivity to menthol of the cold-sensing

nerve-endings which is believed to be at work here. The membranes in the nasal passages feel cooler and as a consequence give a sensation of easier air flow and less congestion.

Peppermint's antiseptic activity

All essential oils are antiseptic to a degree, and peppermint is particularly so, both in direct contact and as a vapour. Dr Jean Valnet, in *The Practice of Aromatherapy*[22], lists in decreasing order the potency of aromatic essences in combating the development of germs and killing them. As a vapour, it comes in tenth place after lemon, thyme, orange, bergamot, juniper, clove, citronella, lavender, and niaouli. If peppermint oil comes into direct contact with bacteria, its antiseptic properties are even greater, only thyme, lemon and juniper having a stronger effect.

In laboratory experiments, essence of peppermint killed staphylococcus, a micro-organism which can infect cuts, causing pus, and which is also often a culprit in food poisoning, in $3^1/2$ hours[22]. It also neutralised the bacillus responsible for tuberculosis[22] and was indeed used at one time in treating this once-prevalent disease.

On a more mundane level, peppermint's antiseptic properties are a useful extra in combating germs in intestinal disorders, in particular diarrhoea and in conditions, like colds, where the respiratory tract is affected. It is reported to have some use as a *vermifuge*, helping to expel intestinal worms[22].

Peppermint and the mind

Peppermint is described in aromatic herbal medicine as a cephalic, an oil whose fragrance influences states of mind.

The sense of smell is triggered by the olfactory cells in the upper part of the nasal cavity, which are linked to the brain.   Each cell has what are known as olfactory hairs which detect odours in the air, stimulate the cells, initiating the sensory pathway by which the brain identifies and reacts to smells.

Smell is controlled by the same area of the brain, the limbic system, that is involved in memory function, learning and emotion, and Robert Tisserand in *Aromatherapy for Everyone*[36] says that there are several ways in which smell and the memory are linked. Claims that certain essential oils have the capacity to stimulate memory and concentration can be traced back to the 1st century AD, he says. The most potent cephalic essences are rosemary, in particular, and also basil and peppermint.

Physiologists at the University of Cincinnati carried out experiments in which whiffs of peppermint were shown to improve alertness in carrying out repetitive tasks by up to 30%[37]. Their findings are borne out by work at another American academic centre, Washington's Catholic University, where the patterns of brainwaves associated with alertness were measured in people who had sniffed peppermint. The sensory pathway for visual detection was reported as being enhanced by the oil's fragrance[37].

Peppermint as a tonic

Tonic is a broad term which applies to many herbal remedies which have a range of pharmacological effects. Peppermint is an excellent example with its action on the digestive system and liver function and its mildly stimulating effect on circulation.

Peppermint as an anti-oxidant

Among recent scientific research into peppermint and approximately 50 other plant extracts has been a series of experiments investigating their anti-oxidant - anti-decaying - properties[38].

The work started in Scotland at the Scottish Agricultural College, and is involving a growing number of other European academic and medical institutions. The Scottish Agricultural College's Auchincruive centre, occupying an extensive former private estate near Ayr in the south-west of Scotland, has a flourishing herb garden, part of a long-term project to establish which herbs will grow so far north and to investigate potential commercial uses for them. Plant extracts with anti-oxidant properties could have a use in the food industry as preservatives, for instance.

Tests at a Hungarian university, in association with the Scottish college, have also found that thyme, the most potent of the anti-oxidant plants, fed to rats and mice, had the ability to slow down the ageing process. Ageing involves the reduction of polyunsaturated fatty acids in the cells, but in animals that were fed the plant extracts the levels remained high, particularly in the liver. Two of the next stages in the research will be to investigate whether the plant extracts can make a significant impact in mitigating the effects of ageing in humans, such as severe memory loss, and to pin-point which chemical constituents in the plants possess the anti-oxidant properties.

Peppermint, according to microbiologist Dr Stan Deans, who heads the Scottish research team, is only 80-90% as effective as thyme as an anti-oxidant, so it will not be one of the extracts to be studied in a programme of clinical trials with humans at various European centres. The programme will take from three to 10 years, depending on the level of funding, if any, from a European Community grant, which at the time of writing the researchers have applied for.

It is certainly premature to recommend a "cup of peppermint tea a day to keep old age at bay", but any new light thrown on the chemistry of a plant with a long record of medicinal use is exciting, and this work is making an important contribution towards a fuller understanding of peppermint's action on the human body.

Questions of safety and toxicity

Peppermint is a drug, and as drugs go it is a pretty safe one. But as with any substance which has positive pharmacological effects on the body, it also has the potential to do harm if not used responsibly, so follow manufacturers' dosage recommendations and keep it out of the reach of children (it wouldn't take long for children, let loose with a 10ml bottle of peppermint oil, to make themselves extremely sick).

Doctors usually regard peppermint oil in prescribed dosages as having a comparatively low risk of serious side effects for most patients; that is why it is so useful in treating irritable bowel syndrome. Anyone with ulcerative colitis or paralytic ileus (a condition of the small intestine) should use it with some caution, though, because it could be irritating. Medical herbalists may be even more cautious and would advise against using peppermint in certain other circumstances, especially in self-treatment.

What is the difference between oil and tincture or infusion of peppermint?

Oil of peppermint is a stronger medicine than a tincture or an infusion. In a tincture, which is made by steeping the herb in alcohol and water at room temperature for a long period, or in an infusion, in which the herb is left in boiling water for a short time, the constituents from watery parts of the plant are retained, as well as those from the oil. During distillation, watery constituents are lost, but as peppermint's medicinal properties are found mainly in the oil, it makes it a more concentrated remedy. Peppermint oil reaches the bloodstream when massaged into the skin, as well as when it is taken as an internal medicine. Inhaling it affects the central nervous system and respiratory passages.

Contraindications and side effects

A proposal for a monograph on peppermint produced by the European Scientific Co-operative for Phytotherapy[26] says that no adverse effects from long-term use of peppermint oil, within recommended levels, are known. It gives average daily doses as 0.2-0.4ml (0.6ml-1.2ml in irritable bowel syndrome). Sometimes peppermint oil is quantified in milligrams, rather than millilitres; 1ml of oil equals between 897mg and 910mg.

Medical herbalist Rosalind Blackwell prescribes peppermint only for a month at a time before allowing a break of at least two weeks. In patients with high blood pressure she would avoid the oil, except for occasional one-off doses, and would be cautious about prescribing it to epilepsy sufferers (if these conditions affect you, ask the advice of your doctor or of a qualified herbal practitioner before using peppermint in self-treatment on a regular basis). She uses it only externally and in great moderation for pregnant women - but do not panic if you are pregnant and have been using it, for the risk is small. But another type of mint, pennyroyal, which was a traditional abortion-inducing herb and contains, in much larger amounts then peppermint, a uterine-stimulating substance called pulegone (a ketone), could be extremely harmful. Peppermint tea in moderation is fine for morning sickness. Peppermint was traditionally reputed to dry milk in nursing mothers, so use with caution during breastfeeding.

As it is a stimulant, taking peppermint late in the

evening might interfere with sleep. Extended use of peppermint is sometimes also reported to cause headaches.

Heartburn can be a result of peppermint causing regurgitation of acid and irritating the upper gastrointestinal tract, the gullet.

Anyone with achlorhydria, a condition which affects the acid balance of their stomachs, should use only enteric-coated capsules[26]. It is also advisable to consult a practitioner if you have bile duct obstruction, gallstones or gall bladder inflammation before using peppermint[26].

Whole peppermint extract - ie tea or tincture - is best avoided by people with peptic or duodenal ulcers, as the bitters it contains stimulate the gastric juices.

Ketones, of which peppermint contains several, are potentially damaging to the nervous system, but there are many different types, some far more toxic than others (those with smallest molecules are the most dangerous). Menthone, the main ketone in peppermint, is one of the least toxic and is present in minute quantities. Consumption would have to be on a massive scale to cause any problems.

Peppermint can occasionally cause severe irritation and rashes in sensitive people, especially if used on the skin, so be cautious when applying it externally[39]. Protect your eyes, as the strong vapours of peppermint can irritate them, let alone direct contact with the oil.

Overdose levels

The ESCOP monograph puts overdose levels of peppermint at 4g (around 3.6ml). Resulting symptoms could be a general sensation of cold, stomach-ache, cardiac problems, ataxia (the inability to co-ordinate muscles in voluntary movement) and other central nervous system problems[40 41 42].

Reports of abuse with peppermint and menthol are

unusual, but should be noted; adverse reactions can result from inhalation. A 13-year-old bronchial asthma sufferer with nasal catarrh was found by his mother, barely rousable and talking gibberish, after inhaling an estimated 5ml instead of the recommended few drops of a preparation containing several ingredients, including menthol and peppermint oil. The menthol was blamed for his temporary, but severe, central nervous system disturbance[41].

Can peppermint be used with children?

If using the oil topically, apply in extremely dilute amounts in an ointment (1 drop in a 60g pot of ointment). For internal use give only peppermint tea, and then in moderation. Do not apply peppermint oil to the nose of babies and small children because of the risk of laryngeal and bronchial spasms[26].

Does peppermint interact with other drugs or herbal remedies?

It should be avoided when receiving homoeopathic treatment, not because it will do any harm, but because it may interfere with the homoeopathic healing process.

Is it advisable to take other essential oils internally?

Peppermint oil has a long history of internal use, but as a rule it is not recommended to take most essential oils internally.

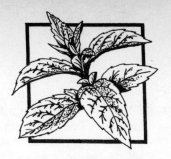

CHAPTER FOUR

Peppermint and irritable bowel syndrome

Oil of peppermint is a classic example of a traditional remedy that has been rediscovered by modern medicine. Today it is recognised as a useful treatment in the common and often chronic digestive disorder of irritable bowel syndrome both by orthodox doctors and by practitioners of herbal medicine.

What makes peppermint's current use in IBS such a good story is that the clinical experience and research by doctors treating the syndrome since the 1970s has brought confirmation and modern scientific credibility for one of its main historic medicinal uses. To describe peppermint as a major breakthrough in the treatment of irritable bowel syndrome would be succumbing to excess literary licence. It does not cure, but it does give considerable relief from the most painful symptoms for many sufferers.

For today's gastroenterologists and GPs, oil of peppermint has added another string to their bow in treating a complicated disorder, which although benign and posing no long-term risk to physical health, is notoriously difficult to treat appropriately. A particular merit of peppermint oil, which has been licensed for prescription on the

National Health Service since the early 1980s, is its low
risk of side effects.

Irritable bowel syndrome - a modern epidemic

Recognition of irritable bowel syndrome as a specific condition has come about in the past 30 years or so. Only in
the last decade has it become widely accepted as a gen-
uine medical problem that can certainly hamper normal
life, can be painful and distressing and affects millions of
people in the UK alone.

The British Digestive Foundation describes irritable
bowel syndrome as an epidemic[43] with up to one in three
British people suffering from it. Some recent research into
the prevalence of IBS carried out among 1,620 patients
from lists of a number of GPs, published in the British
Medical Journal[44], produced more conservative estimates
of around a quarter of the population being affected. But
whether one in three or one in four, it still represents a
huge number of people, so that it is not surprising that
IBS is the most common digestive condition for which
patients seek medical advice.

Typical of gastroenterologists is consultant Dr Douglas
Holdstock, who estimates that two-thirds of his outpatients are irritable bowel sufferers referred by their GPs.
Yet specialists such as Dr Holdstock see only a percentage
of the IBS sufferers who turn up in local doctors' surg-
eries, and not even GPs see the majority of those affected.
In two out of three cases it seems that people never seek
professional medical advice about the condition . . . they
grin and bear it, or treat themselves.

Despite the fact that in many households, in offices, at
parties and within any kind of social setting, statistically
there are likely to be one or several IBS sufferers, it is still
not a "household name" condition. "Irritable bowel what?"
is not an untypical reaction. It is confused with other

digestive problems like colitis or inflammatory bowel disease, which have similar symptoms. Constipation, diarrhoea, tummy rumbles and uncontrollable wind are some of the symptoms of this disorder, sometimes graphically referred to as tense tummy or windy bowel. Hardly surprising, then, that it makes an unlikely topic for general conversation. Many sufferers who have only mild, occasional symptoms are probably not even aware that they are experiencing irritable bowel.

If patients have been reluctant to discuss their IBS, it has to be said that the attitude of some GPs in the past may not always have been encouraging . . . mainly because the condition has been poorly understood. Many doctors would themselves admit that at one time they tended to regard IBS more as a state of mind than as a state of the digestive system.

That attitude has changed during the past decade as the work of hospital specialists has been disseminated through a significant number of reports in medical journals to those working at the sharp end of general practice.

At a popular level, too, IBS is receiving an increasing amount of publicity with an overwhelming response from people who want information and help. The extent of the interest was brought home to the British Digestive Foundation, a charitable body which raises funds for research into digestive disorders and diseases, by the size of its postbag following two pieces of publicity in early 1992. A two-minute breakfast television spot broadcast and a short article in the *Daily Telegraph* both mentioned a booklet on IBS available from the Foundation, whose London offices were inundated with an average 400 requests per day for copies.

How do I know if I have irritable bowel syndrome?

As the description *syndrome* suggests, the condition

encompasses a spectrum of symptoms which may be present in various combinations and various degrees of severity.

The main symptoms are:

> Colicky abdominal pain, usually low down on the left
>
> Pain relieved by a bowel action or the passing of wind
>
> A bloated and windy feeling, sometimes accompanied by rumbling noises
>
> Diarrhoea, particularly around breakfast time
>
> Constipation which may exacerbate the abdominal pain
>
> Irregular bowels alternating between diarrhoea and constipation
>
> Small, hard, pellety stools, like rabbit droppings
>
> Passing mucus with the stools or passing mucus on its own

Not every IBS sufferer experiences *all* these symptoms, but it is unusual for people with other types of disorder to suffer more than two or three of them together. In some people problems are intermittent and a minor inconvenience; in the worst cases sufferers have little respite and the pain is crippling.

Its onset is usually in young or middle adulthood, and although it may disappear for periods it is often recurrent throughout life and may persist into old age. There are several different patterns of symptoms, the most commonly experienced form being irritable or spastic colon in which episodes of abdominal pain and irregular bowel habits are the predominant characteristics.

What has made IBS such a difficult condition to define is that symptoms can involve parts of the body well beyond the digestive system. In women the condition is commonly accompanied by painful periods and intercourse. Other physical symptoms include back pain, headache and sleeping difficulties. In some people the condition may also be linked to mild depression, anxiety, tiredness, panic attacks and emotional disorders. Some sufferers have other problems of the digestive system like heartburn and vomiting, while others may have bowel and bladder disfunction such as frequent passing of urine.

There is more logic to this pattern of symptoms than is immediately apparent, because what they all have in common is control, as of digestion, by the part of the nervous system called the autonomic nervous system, which prompts the body's spontaneous actions. The digestive upset may be part of a wider disruption of the working of this system of nerves. And the underlying cause of it all? Often stress is to blame.

What irritable bowel is not

Because stress is so often bound up with an irritable bowel, a vital part of diagnosis and therapy is simply reassuring patients that their symptoms are not indicative of something far worse.

The good news for anxious patients is that IBS is *not* an organic disease causing any lasting change in the body's structure or tissues. It does not result in inflammation, degeneration or malignancy. Nor does it have links with cancer and other diseases of the bowel such as inflammatory bowel disease, ulcerative colitis or Crohn's disease, although concern that they have got such an illness may cause IBS sufferers hours of unnecessary heartache and worsen their symptoms.

Dr Holdstock explains how stress and worry can create a vicious circle in irritable bowel, especially when it develops in people who are natural worriers. "Perhaps you are stressed - you've got your parents-in-law staying - and you get a bit of tummy ache. If you are a worrying sort of person, you may think 'Oh my goodness, I've got bowel cancer', so you worry more and get another cramp and so it goes on. It's not been proved that such a sequence does happen, but I think it is very likely that it does."

Disconcertingly the symptoms which IBS patients experience are indeed the very kind of symptoms which doctors would expect to be a sign of organic disease, but on further investigation there appears to be nothing physically wrong. It is because of the apparent discrepancy between the patient's subjective description of symptoms and the physical evidence of the doctor's examination that IBS could be dismissed by the unsympathetic doctor as a psychosomatic condition, the product of an over-anxious imagination in patients of a classic neurotic psychological type.

But, says Dr Holdstock, the pain is real, indeed disabling for some people. Irritable bowel sufferers do not make a fuss about nothing.

What does cause the pain and the other symptoms of IBS?

In a nutshell, it is caused by the gastrointestinal tract behaving abnormally. To help explain the problem more fully, a short summary of digestive anatomy and medical terms will be useful.

The gut (also called the gastrointestinal tract or the alimentary canal): This is the muscular tube which propels food from mouth to anus. It includes the gullet (oesophagus), which links the throat (pharynx) to the stomach, the stomach itself, the intestines, large and small, the rectum . . . it's the whole lot.

The bowel: This is the lower part of the gut, the part below the stomach. It includes the *small intestine*, from where most of the nutrients from food, having been thoroughly broken down in the stomach, are absorbed into the bloodstream, and the *large intestine* where the leftover gunge is prepared for dumping . . . during the next visit to the loo.

The colon: This is the major component of the large intestine - our internal waste-processing works.

The gut transports, breaks down and digests food by waves of muscular contractions, technically termed peristalsis. In irritable bowel, the muscle is hyper-sensitive and the rhythm of its contractions is easily upset; too fast and it can cause diarrhoea, too slow and there can be constipation. If the muscle goes into overdrive and produces waves of fierce contractions, particularly in the colon, it produces the griping colicky pains, referred to as spasms, which are familiar to so many irritable bowel sufferers.

These episodes of griping pain are not always entirely due to a sudden spasmodic increase in the rate and fierceness of contraction. If there are retained faeces in the colon or gas trapped in other parts of the bowel, the muscle pressing on it during any contraction probably aggravates the discomfort. The faster the contractions, the more acute the pain.

Why the muscle should be so sensitive is not fully understood, although for some people it may be hereditary or acquired as a result of an illness like gastroenteritis.

Early in the 1960s, when IBS was first being defined, it was thought that only the colon was prone to this sensitivity, and doctors used to talk about irritable colon. In the later '60s, research, in which Dr Holdstock took part, established that the disorder often affected the whole of the bowel, and the latest thinking is that the entire gut may be involved. Indeed, in a few years time doctors will be more likely to talk about irritable gut rather than irritable bowel syndrome.

Just how do nerves and stress come into this?

We tend to think of bowel movements as the most basic, physical function of the body, while our nerves and emotional functioning seem almost abstract. How can one have such a direct effect on the other?

In fact, the nervous system is as physical and mechanical as the digestive system, but on a minute scale . . . its mechanics are those of intricate chemical reactions.

Just such a complex chain of chemical interactions in the nervous and the hormonal systems controls the gut. When we eat and digest food, our body's nervous system knows when to signal to the appropriate part of the gut to start its wave of contractions. As explained in the previous chapter, a nerve originating in the central nervous system sends chemical impulses (neurotransmitters) to every cell in the muscle wall causing contraction or relaxation but, in irritable bowel syndrome, stress disturbs the normal frequency of nervous activity and hence the release of neurotransmitters. The consequence is the slowing down or speeding up of contractions with ensuing digestive mayhem.

Treatment

Treatment can be targeted at various stages of the process which causes irritable bowel symptoms; in practice, doctors may use a combination of two or more of these approaches.

1. In a classic case of irritable bowel clearly provoked by anxiety and characterised by painful spasm of the colon, along with alternate constipation and diarrhoea, ideal treatment would involve combating the underlying stress. Formal psychotherapy or hypnotherapy are ways of tackling the problem, but in practice a doctor is more likely to recommend a yoga class or self-help techniques of relaxation. Occasionally mild anti-depressants are prescribed, but the downside of long-term use of such drugs, with their problems of dependence, hardly needs to be spelt out, and they would usually be used only if other lines of treatment had been unsuccessful.

2. As pain from abnormal muscle contractions is the primary cause of distress in irritable bowel, treatment is often aimed mainly at relieving this particular symptom with what are known broadly as antispasmodic drugs. These fall into two broad categories:

a) anticholinergic drugs which have an indirect antispasmodic action by preventing the effect of the neurotransmitters which trigger spasm. But these drugs can have unpleasant side effects such as dry mouth, dizziness and blurring of vision, a disadvantage which tends to outweigh their benefits in cases of irritable bowel; and

b) straightforward antispasmodics, including oil of peppermint, which act directly on the muscle itself to stop or reduce spasm.

The advantage of oil of peppermint and similar antispasmodics is a low incidence of side effects.

3. A third approach which may go hand-in-hand with other lines of treatment is to regularise bowel habits. Constipation, which also exacerbates the pain of colonic spasm, can be relieved by laxatives or by increasing fibre in the diet. Bulk-forming agents from vegetable sources can also be effective in easing both constipation and diarrhoea. Severe diarrhoea may call for an opium-type drug like codeine, which acts on the brain to modify contractions in the bowel.

Peppermint as an antispasmodic

Calcium plays an important role in regulating contractions of all the body's smooth muscle, including that of the bowel, and during a contraction the amount of calcium in a cell is increased by a tiny amount. As we have already seen, peppermint's antispasmodic action is attributed to menthol temporarily blocking the channels by which calcium reaches the cells. Without a supply of calcium, the muscle relaxes and no longer squeezes so tightly during the contraction, causing less pressure and pain. Peppermint's relaxing effect on the gut also seems to alleviate urgency of bowel motions.

It is peppermint's antispasmodic effect which has attracted pharmaceutical and orthodox medical interest, but reference to its traditional use for digestive complaints and other recent research suggests that peppermint may work in other ways too in irritable bowel syndrome, reducing flatulence both in the intestines and stomach, acting as a mild antiseptic in diarrhoea, and as an anaesthetic on the stomach wall to relieve nausea and prevent vomiting. (How peppermint works is discussed more fully in Chapter 3.)

Some research with patients

There have been a number of clinical trials with oil of peppermint and irritable bowel syndrome. Not all have found oil of peppermint to be beneficial[45 46], but on balance the results have shown it to be effective in relieving the pain and discomfort associated with the condition for a majority of patients.

1. One of the most recent clinical trials demonstrating the benefits of peppermint in IBS treatment was in Denmark (the results were published in 1988 in the Danish equivalent of *The Lancet*)[47]. Outpatients at two Copenhagen hospitals who had clearly-defined irritable bowel syndrome took part. They had at least two of the following three symptoms:

 a) distension and tummy rumbles,

 b) fits of abdominal pain,

 c) varying frequency of motions and/or varying consistency of the stools without any other proven gastrointestinal sickness.

The trial was a double-blind one, which means that half the patients were treated with peppermint oil in soft gelatin capsules (Obbekjaers) and the remainder with a placebo, which in this case was a capsule of soya bean oil. Both sets of capsules were identical in appearance. Four capsules of 200mg of peppermint oil were taken three times a day half an hour before meals, and the patients were asked to keep a daily record of the severity of their symptoms using a three-point scale - no symptoms, mild, and severe.

Additionally there was a once-a-week evaluation of their over-all condition, registered on a five-point scale (much worse, worse, unchanged, better, much better).

After four weeks of treatment, the researchers found that the symptoms of patients on the peppermint oil had lessened significantly more than those of the group taking the placebo (68% of those on peppermint oil reporting improvement as opposed to 26% of those on the placebo). They concluded that the main effect of the oil was pain relief.

2. The results of a trial at Cardiff's University Hospital of Wales by gastroenterologists Dr John Rhodes and Dr Wyn Rees (later at Hope Hospital, Manchester) and pharmacist Brian Evans was published in the *British Medical Journal* in 1979[48]. It was a double-blind trial comparing the effect of peppermint oil, administered in capsules with what is known as an enteric coating to prevent them being broken down by the digestive system before reaching the colon, with that of a placebo of arachis oil which was dispensed in a container injected with peppermint oil to give off a deceiving pepperminty aroma. The patients were asked to keep a daily record of the severity of abdominal and other symptoms. Again the improvement in the symptoms of the patients taking the peppermint was much more marked than of those on the placebo.

The authors concluded that "Peppermint oil in enteric-coated capsules appears to be an effective and safe preparation for symptomatic treatment of the irritable bowel syndrome".

3. A follow-up to this study was a multicentre trial involving 29 patients, all with typical symptoms of the syndrome from seven hospital centres, who were treated with peppermint oil (Colpermin) or placebo. In 1984 a paper in *The British Journal of Clinical Practice*[49] reported that the results had borne out those of the earlier research. "Peppermint oil is a potent agent for relaxation of smooth muscle. This study confirms previous observations of the beneficial effect of peppermint oil for the treatment of irritable bowel syndrome using patient data from several centres."

4. Another piece of research[50] comparing the efficacy of peppermint oil (Colpermin) over a synthetic antispasmodic drug, mebeverine, found the plant remedy to be equally effective. The double-blind trial involved 14 patients and efficacy of the medications was assessed by patients' diary cards and interviews.

Neither preparations had major side effects, but in this trial two patients on the peppermint oil experienced side effects, one heartburn, one slight tiredness, while three receiving mebeverine reported nausea with loss of appetite in one case, upper gastrointestinal disturbances in another, and increased pressure on the bladder in the third. The assessor expressed a preference for oil of peppermint.

5. Forty patients with IBS were treated for periods of two weeks with either enteric-coated peppermint oil capsules, an anticholinergic antispasmodic (l-hyoscyamine) or placebo. Diary cards and interviews were used to assess the treatment and peppermint oil improved the symptom score, whilst there was no significant change with l-hyoscyamine or placebo. Patients on the peppermint oil said that they felt better, whereas those on the other preparations did not feel significantly improved.

The anticholinergic had more side effects than either peppermint oil or placebo[51].

6. Peppermint oil has also been found useful in relaxing the colon during colonoscopy, a diagnostic procedure during which an endoscope is inserted via the rectum, causing the colon to go into spasm. Two doctors found that spraying oil directly on the endoscope reduced colonic spasm within 30 seconds in each patient they tried it on[52 53].

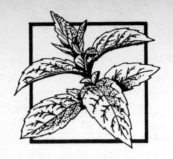

CHAPTER FIVE

Self-treating an irritable bowel with peppermint

Irritable bowel syndrome is a condition which can be safely self-treated . . . as long as you are sure that the symptoms are not due to a more serious problem.

The majority of irritable bowel sufferers never see a doctor about their condition[44] and it seems that those who do are driven to the consulting room, motivated not so much by the degree of their pain and discomfort, but by the level of their anxiety about what the symptoms might signify. Worrying about your symptoms is a good reason in itself for seeking medical advice. Worry can make a sensitive bowel even more irritable, so a reassuring consultation with your GP may settle not only your mind, but also your digestive system.

If your pain and other symptoms are acute and persistent despite self-treatment, then it is always important to see a doctor. Rectal bleeding and dramatic, unexpected weight loss certainly need checking out. In people over 40, IBS-type symptoms, if they are new and persist for more than two or three weeks, can in a few cases be a early sign of bowel cancer.

They could also be due to one of a number of other conditions, most of which are not life-threatening, but which might worsen and cause more pain if not treated appropriately. They may require a different course of treatment from that recommended for irritable bowel.

Seeing your GP does not prevent you treating yourself . . . or consulting a practitioner of herbal medicine. If you are confident that oil of peppermint could help you, you will find products in health food shops and chemists. Alternatively, your doctor may be happy to prescribe it.

Which type of oil of peppermint?

For irritable bowel syndrome you need to take capsules, because they take longer to be broken down and so more of the peppermint reaches the lower bowel.

The oil of peppermint which is prescribed on the NHS is in capsules (called enteric-coated or enterosoluble) specially coated to ensure that they do not break down in the upper digestive system, so all the peppermint is released in the colon rather than absorbed into the blood stream in the small intestine. It also reaches the colon in its original state . . . the process of metabolism has not started to alter the peppermint's chemical composition.

Research comparing enteric-coated preparations (Colpermin) with peppermint in soft gelatin capsules found the former to deliver more unmetabolised peppermint oil to the bowel[55]. However, although the study concluded that the pharmacological effects on the gastrointestinal tract of peppermint in soft gelatin were predominantly in the upper reaches, it suggested that some of the oil probably did nevertheless reach the bowel. This comment is borne out by a double-blind study[47] (reported in Chapter 4) in Denmark using soft gelatin capsules (Obbekjaers) which were found to relieve fits of abdominal pain in nearly 70% of patients.

The researchers in this case concluded that enteric-coating might have had the advantage of reducing the frequency of side effects such as burping and heartburn, which is the result of regurgitated acid from the stomach irritating the gullet. Peppermint can also repeat, so you get a taste of it in your mouth.

Enteric-coated peppermint oil capsules can be bought off-prescription at pharmacies, as well as being prescribed. They contain higher doses of peppermint oil than health food shop brands, but are quite expensive if you do not have a prescription.

Peppermint in other forms, such as tea, tablets or ordinary capsules, seems not to have such a strong, specific action in the colon, but may have a broader effect in the digestive tract. Enteric-coating would work against peppermint's mild anaesthetic action on the stomach, for instance, because it does not get released until further down the digestive tract.

Oil of peppermint as part of a broader treatment

Although oil of peppermint can bring great relief to many sufferers of irritable bowel syndrome, it is not a cure. Its usefulness is in relieving some of the symptoms, rather than eliminating the root cause. The chances of long-term relief are increased if you use oil of peppermint with other approaches.

As has been discussed, stress is often a crucial factor in provoking the problem. Are there clearly identifiable circumstances causing anxiety in your life? Can they be changed? These are the kind of questions which need to be asked if you have IBS.

An extreme means of coping with stress is to take anti-depressants. Hypnotherapy and psychotherapy offer non-drug alternatives, but stress-reduction need not be on such a formal level. Some simple relaxation techniques carried out in the privacy of your home may be just as effective.

Common sense and medical research[55] point to food also playing a part in aggravating the irritability of the bowel, but the relationship between what we eat and what causes the bowel to misfunction is a complicated one. Although some IBS patients, for instance, may be recommended a high-fibre diet to ease constipation, some sufferers find that too many wheat products are part of the cause of their problems and "neat" bran, which is never an ideal way for anyone to increase dietary fibre, may worsen their condition.

Intolerance to various foods is found in IBS patients, but there is no consistent link with any particular products. Different people vary in the way that their digestive system reacts to their diet. As a generalisation, though, foods that are most likely to exacerbate irritable bowel are wheat, corn, dairy products, coffee, oats, rye, tea, citrus fruits, fatty and fried foods, onions, cabbage, salads and alcohol. Smoking can also make the condition worse[56].

Fat may be a heightening factor in irritable bowel. There is some evidence that in IBS sufferers the colon is more sensitive to fat which can help trigger spasms of the the bowel muscles.

Two paperback guides full of practical advice about tackling irritable bowel with changes in eating habits and adjustments to lifestyle are *Coping Successfully with Your Irritable Bowel*[56] and *The Irritable Bowel Diet Book*, both by Rosemary Nicol.

Users' experiences

Looking back, Caroline, 44, can laugh about the time her urgent bowel movements caught her short during what was supposed to be a convivial visit to the pub. At the time, though, it caused her acute embarrassment and was typical of the incidents which were curtailing her social life because they made her nervous about going out.

"This particular time I had to rush to the loo and I was in there for ages, it seemed like an eternity. It was the only loo in the pub and I knew there were people waiting. It was awful. I got to the point with my irritable bowel problems where I was having to do a runner to the loo at least once a week because I had what I call an 'explosion'."

Her GP had prescribed an antispasmodic drug, but although it worked initially it became less effective.

"Having read a lot more on the subject and meeting others with the same problem, I decided to try something else. I found peppermint oil capsules in the health food shop and decided to give them a try.

"The peppermint does seem to help - I don't get the attacks so frequently - and I now take the capsules before I eat at lunchtime and in the evening. Sometimes I found that if I took the capsules after a meal the peppermint would repeat and I'd get a taste of it in my throat."

Caroline, who describes herself as a natural worrier, has also taken up yoga to help her cope with the stress which hits her digestive system so hard. The power of positive thinking has also made a difference. She has found that simply understanding irritable bowel and meeting other people who are affected more severely has given her confidence to carry on with normal socialising. "I refuse to let it worry me now."

Margaret , who is in her 60s, had suffered from irritable bowel syndrome for many years, but had been told by her GP that she would just have to learn to live with it. The fact that he is a man makes it more difficult, she says, to talk about an embarrassing problem.

In retrospect, she can see that she has always had a sensitive digestive system, not helped by her mother's rigorous approach to bowel health, involving regular doses with syrup of figs. But she traces her irritable bowel back particularly to when her son was a demanding, tiny baby,

30 or so years ago, when she frequently repressed bowel movements because it was difficult to get to the lavatory.

Possibly as a reaction, the worst aspect of her irritable bowel has been attacks of urgently needing to go to the loo.

"I was becoming frightened to travel any distance in case I was stricken. The attacks were embarrassing because I never knew when an attack would take place. I've had a number of occasions when I've been in the public library, for instance, and had to get home pronto.

"I read about oil of peppermint in the medical column of a women's weekly. It has helped enormously. It didn't stop the attacks completely, but has greatly reduced the number and severity."

She has since met another irritable bowel sufferer at her bridge club and recommended it to her. Margaret has been taking peppermint oil for six years and has experienced no side effects. She also takes a herbal tranquilliser occasionally to relieve stress.

Mary, 67, read a magazine feature about the benefits of peppermint in irritable bowel problems, from which she had suffered along with diverticulitis (inflammation in the colon).

"It caused great discomfort, pain and a general feeling of embarrassment at certain times when one had to tolerate the noise of a rumbling tummy. It made one feel rather low at times."

Although another antispasmodic preparation prescribed by her doctor had given little relief, she found peppermint oil, taken with the full agreement of her GP, eased the pain and flatulence. The only side effect was a very slight case of repeating after an hour or so, but it was not unpleasant enough to discontinue taking the peppermint.

Sandra, 48, is a long-term sufferer of irritable bowel syndrome. When she first developed a pain in the right-hand side of her stomach, she was desperately worried that she had cancer of the bowel. She missed time at work and was put through a series of invasive, sometimes painful, medical tests, all proving negative.

"I asked a surgeon once what was causing the problem and he said, 'You tell me'!

"The worry made the problem worse and worse. It was mainly the pain, which could be dreadful, and alternately diarrhoea and constipation. Sometimes it caused very bad flatulence.

"Eventually a friend showed me a magazine article about peppermint oil, so I tried it. It has not cured my IBS, but I feel it has certainly helped control it and the pain is not so severe"

Brenda, 78, has suffered from irritable bowel for many years and has always found that peppermint gives relief from digestive problems, especially nervous indigestion.

"I've been taking peppermint since I was a child. My father was a pharmacist and used to make himself and the rest of the family a bedtime drink of oil of peppermint in hot water. If ever we had a tummy ache we would have a dose of peppermint."

*The majority of the case histories were obtained through the UK distributors of Obbekjaers peppermint oil products. Permission to publish the information was given by all the people involved, but in most cases the names have been changed.

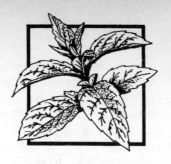

CHAPTER SIX

Peppermint, a remedy for today

Scientific research is enhancing peppermint's credibility as a modern-day remedy; it provides a rationale for some of the ways in which this healing plant has been used in the past and is creating a firm place for it in medicine of the future.

But exciting and encouraging as it is when modern medical investigation provides supporting evidence for the traditional use of a herb, we should not downgrade the value of what can be learned from centuries of observation and written and verbal testimonials telling of successful treatment. They are in themselves often a validation.

Folklore is not just a feature of the past, but is still being added to and passed on today. That many people have memories of peppermint as the remedy that "Granny used to recommend", perhaps for indigestion or for headaches, speaks volumes for peppermint's efficacy. And, as in Granny's day, the relief it brings for all kinds of minor ailments that afflict most families now and again makes it a valuable basic item in any household's first aid kit.

Herbal remedies are on the whole a particularly safe type of medicine. That does not mean that there are no

plants which are poisonous (there are many that are highly toxic even in small amounts, *but* these are not used in
herbal medicines). Nor does it mean that remedies like
peppermint carry no risk if used irresponsibly (see the
section on Safety and Toxicity in Chapter 3).

But herbal remedies usually contain less concentrated
amounts of pharmacological ingredients - substances
which have a medicinal effect - compared to many synthetic medicines based on a single active substance. A
remedy made by extracting ingredients from the whole
plant, like a tincture or an infusion, contains many substances, not just the main medicinal component. These
other constituents modify - dilute, if you like - the remedy's action, making its effect less heavy-handed.

Herbal remedies do sometimes take longer to work,
although this is not always the case. Remember that
although the various component substances act as a
mutual braking system, preventing any individual substance from becoming too powerful, many of them also
have their own medicinal properties, so the remedy is
healing on several fronts. In aromatic herbs, including
peppermint, many of the medicinal attributes are found
mainly in the oil, so when it is separated through the
process of distillation from the watery parts, the end
result is a more medicinally-concentrated substance.

Nevertheless, essential oils like peppermint do not contain a single constituent; they are a mix of various components, all of them have a modifying action on each other.

The main active ingredient of peppermint is menthol,
and if that is extracted from the oil it makes a more powerful and, for some purposes, a highly useful medicinal
substance. But menthol on its own does not have the bal-
ancing breadth of healing properties which is found in
whole oil of peppermint and which makes it a better
product for self-medication.

Forms of peppermint

Whole dried herb can be bought loose or in teabags for making infusions, ie cups of peppermint tea.

Tinctures are alcoholic extracts of the whole plant. Available mainly through herbal practitioners.

Peppermint essential oil comes in various forms: in dropper bottles; as tablets; as powder (which can be made into a hot drink); in ordinary capsules; and in strengthened capsules, known as enteric-coated or enterosoluble.

Traditional preparations such as peppermint emulsion, peppermint water and peppermint spirit are no longer frequently sold, but can be obtained through chemists.

Peppermint's best-known form is probably still as confectionery, and it is real peppermint oil, rather than artificial flavour, that is used in most products. The difference between these and medicinal preparations, however, is the smaller quantity of peppermint needed for flavouring than that required for a pharmacological effect.

How to use oil of peppermint

Oil of peppermint can be used in a number of ways; as an internal treatment, by inhaling it, or externally by rubbing it into or applying it to the skin (in most cases diluted with a vegetable oil). When applied to the skin, essential oils still penetrate into the bloodstream[22].

How much peppermint to use

Oil
Manufacturers of essential oils usually give instructions about amounts to use in various applications, but as a general guide:

For internal use: 1 drop with a teaspoon of honey or, even better, in olive oil. Take with food. With capsules and tablets follow manufacturers' recommendations.

For massage: For most applications peppermint should be diluted, 1-5 drops in 10ml of a base oil (see below). As a general rule in massage with essential oils, most aromatherapists and manufacturers recommend around 5 drops of a single or a blend of oils in 10ml (15 drops in 30ml or 25 drops in 50ml for larger applications), but with peppermint many advise greater dilution because it can irritate the skin. When using peppermint for the first time, under rather than over-estimate the amount needed to be effective.

Base oils should be vegetable (preferably cold-pressed and organic). Suitable oils are grapeseed, which has a light odour, sunflower, soya, peanut, apricot kernel, almond, safflower, hazelnut and corn oil. If storing a blend, add a small amount of wheatgerm oil (10%), which has anti-oxidant properties. For single applications, a 5ml-dose medicine spoon is useful.

For a skin ointment: Add 3 drops of peppermint (1 drop for children) to a 60g jar of calendula or other soothing cream like chickweed, and stir with a sterilised implement. To use on a baby or small child, just one drop of peppermint oil in a 60g pot would be sufficient.

For inhalation: 2-5 drops added to a bowl of hot water (use about a pint) or put drops on to cotton wool (a small bottle with a removable lid will stop the oil from evaporating).

For essential oil diffusers (vaporisers): 4 drops. If you do not own a special diffuser, put the essential oil on a piece of cotton wool and secure it to a radiator in contact with the heat.

For a bath: Use it only in a formula with other oils, around 5 drops in total.

For a footbath: 2-4 drops.

For a handbath: 2-3 drops.

For a mouthwash: 1 drop thoroughly stirred in a pint of water.

For compresses: 3-6 drops in a bowl of water (hot for chronic pain, menstrual cramps and tummy pain, icy cold for headaches). Agitate to disperse the oil, place a flannel on top of the water to soak up the surface oils and then gently squeeze out excess water. Place the compress on the affected area and cover with a dry towel. Leave until the compress has warmed or cooled to body temperature.

Dried
If using dried peppermint in a loose form, you need around 1 teaspoon per cup. Pour on boiling water and leave to steep in a covered container for 5-15 minutes. The longer it is left, the stronger the brew.

   Dried peppermint also comes in teabags, which should be left to steep in boiling water for at least 5 minutes.

Fresh
The required amount to make an infusion from fresh leaves varies tremendously from plant to plant. Soil conditions and the stage of the growing season can affect the potency of the leaves, and even a single leaf of peppermint at certain times of the growing season might make a strong cuppa - you need to experiment. To infuse, chop or gently bruise the leaves and stand them in boiling water for 5-10 minutes.

Storing essential oil

Essential oil should be kept in dark-glass bottles in cool, dry conditions and away from light and air. Secure the tops well because essential oil quickly evaporates when exposed to air.

When to use peppermint

The following A-Z of conditions in which peppermint can be used to excellent effect is a broad-ranging round-up of its potential uses.

Peppermint is not always the only, or even the most obvious, herbal treatment, and in many instances it can be even more beneficial when combined with other herbs. Home medicine cupboards, however, do not necessarily carry a huge range of herbal extracts and since many conditions suitable for self-treatment strike unexpectedly, they have to be dealt with using remedies readily to hand. Peppermint is a useful product to have on standby because of its broad range of uses.

Where peppermint is likely to be more effective used in combination with other herbal extracts, this is indicated.

There are also some conditions listed here which are unsuitable for self-medication, but which a medical herbalist might treat with peppermint probably in conjunction with other herbs. Chapter 7 describes a herbalist's approach to healing and gives information about contacting a practitioner.

For children, use an extremely dilute ointment or give warm, rather than hot, tea (not too hot or too strong) sweetened with honey to drink or to inhale.

Before using peppermint refer to the section on Safety and Toxicity in Chapter 3.

With all self-treatment, if symptoms persist seek medical advice.

ACHES AND PAINS

Part of the traditional herbal approach to conditions involving inflammation is to rub into the skin substances, including volatile oils such as peppermint, which dilate the underlying blood vessels, so increasing the inflammatory effect. This inflammation, an increase in blood flow, is seen as the body's way of coping with injury or irritation, rather than a problem in itself, because it is carrying elements such as white blood cells which help repair and cleanse the affected area.

Peppermint can be used on its own in a base of vegetable oil for topical pain relief or application in a warm compress. For an even more invigorating massage oil for the relief of aches and pains in muscles, joints and nerves caused by sporting injury or conditions such as rheumatism, arthritis, lumbago and sciatica, put into a 30ml bottle:

    3 drops of peppermint
    4 drops each of lavender, rosemary, and juniper
    Top up with a base vegetable oil.

For a **pre-sports rub** to increase circulation to the muscles, blend peppermint with rosemary.

For a **sprained ankle** try the hot and cold treatment. You need two bowls, one with water as cold as you can stand it containing 2 or 3 drops of oil of peppermint, the other with hot water and 2 or 3 drops of oil of rosemary. Place the ankle alternately in each bowl. If there seems any possibility of a fracture, get medical attention.

Two effective herbal remedies for rubbing into sprains are comfrey and witch hazel.

Use
Oil diluted in base oil.

Users' experiences
A fellow yoga teacher recommended peppermint in massage oil to 54-year-old Janette after she experienced stiff-

ness in her knee and ankle joints. Positive thinking makes Janette reluctant to dwell on a suspicion that she may have a touch of arthritis. Although her discomfort was not particularly affecting everyday movement, during yoga sessions she was finding it difficult to hold certain postures, such as the lotus position, for any length of time.

"After a particularly strenuous session I was experiencing aching and tired ankles and knees. Descending stairs, my knees gave clicking sounds and sometimes I experienced a certain degree of stiffness," says Janette, who is an experienced yoga practitioner.

After rubbing peppermint oil round her knees and ankles daily Janette's movement increased and strenuous yoga classes no longer left her aching. She also found that paying special attention to the diet, such as cutting out sweets and chocolate, further improved her condition, but when she stopped applying the oil the stiffness and aching returned.

Arthritis of the spine means that 85-year-old Margaret suffers regular pain, running from her hip to the back of the neck. She cannot walk without pain and has been housebound for five years. Paracetamol is her only other pain relief.

"I have tried several things, but always go back to oil of peppermint which eases the pain whenever I use it. I felt it was so good I even sent a bottle to my daughter in Australia."

Mrs S rubs oil of peppermint into her arm to relieve the pain of tennis elbow. "The pain was stopping me from knitting and sewing, but rubbing in the oil gives great relief."

Mrs P, who is in her 80s, says that she has come to rely on peppermint oil to give periods of respite from the pain of

arthritis in her spine and her hips, usually using it in preference to pain-killing drugs.

"Pain-killers never achieved very much, unless I took
very strong ones in which case there was the problem of
side effects. Rubbing peppermint oil on the painful parts
gives me temporary respite and therefore a chance to
sleep, if applied late at night."

As a small child in the years before 1918 she remembers
her grandmother taking peppermint for indigestion . . .
"and also if she felt a bit out of sorts she would take it.
Peppermint was quite current then."

In contrast, during a recent spell in hospital Mrs P
pleaded for three hours for peppermint to relieve indigestion. "I managed to get one dose, but I think the request
was considered eccentric." She usually takes a daily peppermint capsule, feeling that it has a general tonic effect.

ARTHRITIS

Use peppermint oil in a massage oil singly or in combination with other essential oils to rub into the affected area
for pain relief (see Aches and pains above).

A number of people who have used oil of peppermint
as an internal treatment for other conditions report relief
from arthritis as an unexpected benefit.

There is nothing in the properties of peppermint to suggest that it will have a major direct effect on the inflammation of rheumatoid arthritis. Its tonic, invigorating
properties may provide part of the explanation, because
by improving general well-being they make pain easier to
cope with.

Another possibility lies in the stomach and the link
between rheumatoid arthritis and intolerance to foods,
particularly milk, according to writer Barbara Griggs, in
an article on mint published in *Country Living* magazine[37].
She points to the plant's traditional use of aiding the
digestion of milk and suggests that if mint really can

improve digestive efficiency, its use against arthritis deserves more investigation.

Stimulating circulation is part of the traditional herbal approach to arthritic disease. It also emphasises the need for improving bowel and liver function as part of enhancing all aspects of the body's digestive and eliminatory systems. Peppermint does help on both these fronts.

Herbalism, however, offers a much broader approach using a combination of plants, including peppermint in some cases, selected to suit the individual. A medical herbalist can advise - see Chapter 7.

Use
Oil in tablets, capsules or powder.

User's experience
A woman in her 70s takes peppermint oil in capsules to alleviate the pain of osteoarthritis in her knees.

"I started taking them about four years ago after hearing about them from a telephone repairman. I'd remarked about how agile he was and he told me had got arthritis in the knees, but had been helped by taking peppermint oil. I tried them and after a while found a great benefit. They do keep me relatively free from the pains in the knees, although kneeling still is a bit of a problem. I did stop taking them for a short while and tried cod liver oil, because it was a bit cheaper, but as I began to have more pain in the knees again I went back on to the peppermint."

ASTHMA
Peppermint's expectorant action, helping to expel the mucus from the bronchial tubes, makes it useful as an inhalant. It is not a substitute for professional medical treatment and should be used in moderation.

Use
Inhale oil, 2-5 drops in a bowl of hot water.

BRONCHITIS
Used as an inhalant, peppermint can help relieve congestion through its expectorant action (see Asthma above).

Use
Inhale oil, 2-5 drops in a bowl of hot water.

CATARRH AND SINUSITIS
Inhaling peppermint makes the nasal passages feel less congested. Either make a steam inhalation or drink peppermint tea. A hot drink can also be made from peppermint oil powder.
   To make an inhalation add to a bowl of hot water:
   1 drop of peppermint oil
   2 drops of eucalyptus
   2 drops of rosemary
A drop or two of the oils can also be sprinkled on a pillow to aid sleep at night; if you are a restless sleeper, add soothing lavender.

Use
Oil to inhale, or drink tea.

CHILBLAINS
See Circulation below.

CIRCULATION
Peppermint gently stimulates blood flow, so aiding circulation. It is one of many herbs known as peripheral vasodilators, some of which are used in clinical practice as part of the treatment in conditions where circulation is poor, like arteriosclerosis, Raynaud's disease and Buerger's disease[27].

Serious problems such as this obviously require professional attention (herbs most used to treat circulatory problems in professional herbalism include prickly ash, ginger
and capsicum). Self-treatment with peppermint could help,
however, in cases where circulation is generally poor and
causing problems like chilblains (inflamed, irritating patches on the extremities, toes, fingers, nose, ears), cramps, restless legs, or cold hands and feet. In cases of cold feet due to
bad circulation, a lotion or massage oil containing peppermint oil can be massaged in directly, the massage itself
aiding circulation as well as the absorbed oil.

There is some anecdotal evidence of relief from varicose veins after using peppermint internally. Varicose
veins are a result of bad circulation, but with the compli-
cation of a number of factors including weakness in the
walls of the blood vessels, which makes them less effective in pumping blood back to the heart against the pull of
gravity. Overweight and constipation contribute to the
problem, and people who spend a lot of time standing are
particularly at risk because the blood in their legs finds it
more difficult to circulate.

Peppermint is not a conventional herbal treatment in
this condition although its gentle stimulating effect on circulation may help. Whether you already have varicose
veins or want to prevent them, peppermint in a footbath
is an excellent treatment for tired feet and legs, or apply it
in a lotion or massage oil. Always use upward strokes to
encourage blood flow towards the heart. Avoid vigorous
massage with varicose veins.

Use
Oil in capsules, tablets, powder, massage oil or lotion.

Users' experiences
Dulcie Hollins, who is now in her 60s, has suffered from
poor circulation since childhood. She has used herbal and

other alternative forms of medicine throughout her life and started taking peppermint a few years ago after seeing an advertisement in a chemist shop window.

"Each winter as a child I experienced severe chilblains on both feet and at one time had to have medical treatment. As an adult I still suffered at times with chilblains, and my feet particularly, but also my hands, were constantly extremely cold. It makes one's life quite miserable. I now take peppermint pills usually from the end of September until about April each year, just one a day. My circulation has greatly improved and I would not be without them."

A woman in her 60s took peppermint oil for three years for poor circulation.

"I always felt cold even in warm weather. I found it quite beneficial whilst I was taking it. I did tell my doctor that I was taking it and he said if it helped my condition to continue. I stopped taking it because as I suffer from angina and am seen at the local hospital every three months, I have to take several types of tablets, so I felt I had enough medication."

Ejgil Gronholdt, a state-registered chiropodist from Praesto in Denmark, has recommended peppermint powder (Obbekjaers) to patients with circulation problems for many years.

"A married couple who came to me . . . told me of their experience in the use of peppermint. The wife was being driven mad by her husband's nocturnal tramping around the floor of their house. He suffered terribly from leg cramps at night. He was a retired French cook and had a violent temperament, so that it was no quiet matter when he wanted to get up and tramp around the house in the middle of the night. They had tried a number of different remedies . . . but none of them gave any relief."

Mr Gronholdt gave them some peppermint powder and within a month the couple reported that the night cramps had disappeared, as had the man's bad breath. His morning cough was also much less severe.

COLDS AND FLU

By encouraging sweating, peppermint's heating effect helps bring the temperature down. It is commonly used in colds and flu with elderflowers and yarrow. Infuse dried elderflowers and yarrow and add dried peppermint or a drop of peppermint oil.

To make a cold treatment mixture, combine equal quantities of the dried herbs and use 1-2 teaspoons per cupful.

Sniffing peppermint will also dry a runny nose.

As **prevention**, put peppermint's antiseptic properties to good use in an essential oil diffuser in homes and offices where there are cold and flu germs.

Use
Tea, powder or a drop of oil in a hot drink.

COLD SORES

Peppermint is reputed to have anti-viral properties. For cold sores (caused by the herpes virus) dab a drop of oil neat on to the affected area. (Not for use in genital herpes.)

Use
Oil drops.

COLIC

Colic is griping pain caused by spasm of the bowel, especially in the colon, and can be part of the irritable bowel syndrome. Use peppermint oil in capsules. Also try a warm compress. In a one-off attack, take peppermint immediately. In chronic cases, follow manufacturers' recommended dosages.

Use
Oil in capsules.

Caution: Persistent symptoms may indicate a more serious underlying problem and warrant medical advice.

CONSTIPATION
Peppermint is not a laxative in the conventional sense, but it can relieve constipation due to a sluggish liver. The way that the bowel is working is often connected to the state of the liver, which produces the body's natural laxative, bile[57] and peppermint has bile-stimulating (cholagogue) properties.

Use
Tea or oil in capsules, tablets or powder.

User's experience
Elizabeth suffered chronic constipation until reading about peppermint oil in a magazine. "I took my first tablet immediately after a Sunday lunch and by teatime I was transformed. I have taken one tablet after each meal ever since."

DIARRHOEA
Peppermint relaxes bowel contractions and also has a mild antiseptic effect.

Use
Oil in capsules.

DYSPEPSIA
This is a digestive disturbance, characterised by nausea, heartburn, stomach congestion or discomfort and vomiting. Causes may simply be overindulgence in food and drink, or the symptoms may indicate irritable bowel syn-

drome. For mild indigestion after over-eating or drinking too much, try a cup of peppermint tea or peppermint oil in capsule, tablet or other form. Alternatively take a drop of oil of peppermint with a drop of dill and a drop of fennel in a cup of hot water, sweetened with honey.

Use
Tea or oil

Caution: Persistent dyspepsia can be a sign of more serious illness, so in this case seek medical advice.

ECZEMA
See Skin problems.

FLATULENCE
For wind in the stomach . . .

Use
A drop of oil of peppermint and a drop of oil of fennel plus a teaspoonful of honey in a cup of hot water. Or peppermint oil in tablets, capsules or powder.

. . . and for wind in the intestines. . .

Use
Oil in capsules.

Caution: Use tea if pregnant.

GENERAL WELL-BEING
As a general tonic peppermint can stimulate a sense of well-being.

Use
Oil or tea

User's experience

An 83-year-old widow had a number of health problems, including sleeplessness and an acid stomach, tracing back to her husband's death 10 years before.

"As we were very happy I was distraught, badly needed a shoulder to cry on and was lonely. The doctor said there was nothing wrong and gave me some pain-killers, but this gave me no relief. I took vitamin C as a pick-me-up until I discovered oil of peppermint when I picked up a booklet in a health food shop. It's a wonderful helpmate for sleeplessness, I don't suffer from that any more and it clears the sinuses. When I feel miserable I take a cup with two drops in it to sip. It seems to make life worth living."

HEADACHES AND MIGRAINE

Use the oil externally, dotting it on the temples and ear lobes, neat or combined with lavender. Alternatively use a cold compress. If the headache is a result of a digestive upset, take peppermint internally.

Use

Oil drops applied externally, or take tea or oil in capsule, tablet, or powder form.

HEARTBURN

Some people report relief from heartburn with peppermint, and oil of peppermint is licensed for treating this condition in Denmark. Use with caution, however, because heartburn is often found to be a side effect of peppermint.

Use

Tea or oil in tablets or powder.

HIATUS HERNIA

Some of the digestive upsets caused by hiatus hernia, a

condition in which the stomach wall muscle protrudes through the diaphragm, may be relieved by peppermint. Slippery elm is another herbal remedy which is particularly recommended, before and after meals.

Use
Oil rather than tea, as bitters in the whole herb are not recommended because they stimulate gastric juices.

User's experience
76-year-old Mrs N started taking peppermint after writing for a free sample advertised in a health magazine and has found it helps reduce the discomfort associated with her hiatus hernia.

"The first time I took it was for a very bad tummy ache and it gave immediate relief. I continued to take it and found it helped prevent the pain that I sometimes get after eating something, I suppose it is trapped wind. It's a terrible pain when you get it, but I find I suffer a lot less if I take peppermint regularly."

IRRITABLE BOWEL SYNDROME
Peppermint is useful for a number of the symptoms associated with this digestive disorder, and is particularly beneficial for the griping pain caused by spasm in the bowel. See Chapters 4 and 5.

INDIGESTION
See Dyspepsia.

LIVER DISORDERS
Peppermint is a useful herb in treating liver disorders, but only under medical supervision.

One of the less serious manifestations of sluggish liver function is constipation (see under relevant entry).

MENTAL FATIGUE

Peppermint is what is known as a cephalic - its aroma seems to have an effect on the brain. To aid alertness during work and for a mild, uplifting effect after mental fatigue, burn a few drops of peppermint oil on an essential oil diffuser. Robert Tisserand recommends it particularly for confusion and indecision[8]. Peppermint will probably be most effective if used occasionally in this way, rather than routinely.

Use
Drops of oil singly or in combination with rosemary or basil.

MORNING SICKNESS

All herbs should be treated with caution in pregnancy (see the section on Safety and Toxicity in Chapter 3).

Avoid peppermint *oil* in pregnancy unless given under professional medical supervision, but an infusion or tea can be used in moderation and is particularly effective against morning sickness. The oil could be used as an inhalation to check nausea - a couple of drops in a bowl with boiling water.

Use
Oil drops as inhalant, or tea.

MOSQUITO REPELLENT

Put a drop of oil of peppermint behind the ears or on the wrist, but use cautiously to test the skin's sensitivity and dilute if necessary. Can also be used in combination with citronella and spike lavender.

Use
Neat or diluted oil.

MOUTHWASH
One or two drops of peppermint diluted in a pint of water makes an antiseptic mouthwash. Shake well to disperse or add to 2.5-5ml of vodka then dissolve.

Use
Oil.

NAUSEA
Peppermint has an anaesthetic effect on the stomach wall, so quelling nausea and the desire to vomit.

Use
Tea or oil in tablets, capsules or powder.

PAINFUL PERIODS
Periods can provoke an irritable bowel, leading to spasms in the gut.

Use
Oil in capsules. Also try a warm compress. Herbalists also use peppermint in combination with other herbs in hormone-related menstrual disturbances.

PROSTATE PROBLEMS
Peppermint can help in benign enlargement, especially in the early stages, but this is a problem which always requires professional medical help.

PRURITIS
See Skin problems.

PSORIASIS
See Skin problems.

SCIATICA
See Massage.

SKIN PROBLEMS

The cool sensation of peppermint when the oil is applied to the skin helps relieve itching, while its antiseptic properties counter infection in skin problems such as eczema, pruritus, urticaria and psoriasis. Always use diluted in oil or ointment and with caution in case it causes irritation (for instructions in making a peppermint ointment, see How much peppermint to use, at the beginning of this chapter).

To relieve itching in eczema, also add 2-4 drops of anti-inflammatory chamomile (chamomile matricaria, *not* chamomile maroc) to a 60g jar.

Use
Oil in dilution.

Users' experiences

Herbalist Carol Church's young daughter was smothered in a rash after pulling up handfuls of a garden weed alkanet. She had been wearing shorts and everywhere she had been exposed was red and swollen. Various treatments were tried to no effect, including calamine lotion and chamomile, but a dilution of one drop of peppermint oil in 100ml of water applied to her skin cleared it overnight.

Ejgil Gronholdt, the Danish chiropodist (see Circulation) recommends a peppermint ointment (Obbekjaers, not yet available in this country) to patients with skin problems.

"One lady of 50 has had poliomyelitis (a paralysing disease of the nervous system) for most of her life. Her feet are very deformed and she has overlying toes, which have produced hard skin and corns in many places. The frequent application of peppermint ointment to the exposed places has helped this patient in a quite fantastic way, whereas she has not previously noted any positive effect, in spite of her using a long series of products."

In the case of someone suffering from psoriasis: "He has received comfort by smearing peppermint ointment all the way round his scalp and on his forearms and other typical points of attack on the body. He has not been completely cured, but has obtained considerable relief."

Mr Gronholdt's own father had an eczema-type complaint for which he consulted a skin specialist for several years. "Peppermint ointment was the only remedy that had a beneficial effect on the irritating ulcerations which continually appeared." Mr Gronholdt also notes peppermint's effectiveness against cold sores.

A doctor writing in an American medical journal[58] about pruritis, a condition characterised by a sensation of itching caused by a range of underlying problems, suggests a topical application of menthol in a dilution of 0.25% or 0.5% to give temporary relief.

SHINGLES
To give pain relief, use 2-5% maximum of peppermint oil in a blend with St John's Wort oil, which also has pain-relieving properties.

Use
Diluted oil.

SPORTS INJURIES
See Massage.

TOOTHACHE
Massage oil into the cheek near the painful tooth.

Use
Drops of oil topically.

TRAVEL SICKNESS
Take peppermint tablets at regular intervals during a journey, but not exceeding the manufacturer's recommended amount. Alternatively dab a drop of peppermint on a hanky to inhale, or add a pinch of ginger powder to peppermint tea.

Use
Tea or oil, as drops to inhale, or in tablets.

VARICOSE VEINS
See Circulation.

*The majority of the case histories were supplied through the UK distributors of Obbekjaers peppermint oil products. Permission to publish the information was given by all the people involved, but in most cases the names have been changed.

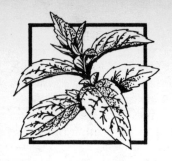

CHAPTER SEVEN

Peppermint in practice

If you want to be treated by specialists in plant medicines, the area of medicine to turn to is medical herbalism.

Herbalism's most evident distinguishing feature is its use of the extracts of roots, leaves, stems and seeds of plants as healing agents, rather than synthetic drugs. Medical herbalists also tend not to use plant medicines to treat only symptoms, but prefer to apply them in such a way that they encourage the body's own healing processes.

A particular type of plant extract, the essential oils of aromatic plants, are also used in aromatherapy. In the UK the therapy's main approach is to massage the oils into the body so that they are absorbed through the skin, but they can also be inhaled or used in the bath and, as the name aromatherapy suggests, the fragrance of the oils contributes to their effect. Aromatherapy is widely perceived in this country as being quite a separate form of treatment from herbalism; aromatherapists work with essential oils while medical herbalists usually use other types of plant extracts such as tinctures and infusions. The distinction is an artificial one and it is more precise to describe aromatherapy as a specialist area of herbal medicine and essential oils as one type of herbal remedy.

It is the case that traditionally, British herbalists have tended not to prescribe essential oils as much as other forms of herbal medicines or to be specifically trained in their use. This is not the case with their colleagues in other countries such as France, where essential oils are widely used by conventional doctors, as well as by alternative practitioners.

Rosalind Blackwell, a medical herbalist and practitioner in aromatic medicine, is helping to bridge the gap between British medical herbalism and aromatherapy. She is unusual in British medical herbalist circles in that not only is she qualified in the more conventional forms of herbalism, but she also spent time in France studying aromatic medicine and learning about the medical application of essential oils, including their uses as internal medicines. She prescribes essential oils, including peppermint, extensively to her patients, using various forms: capsules, inhalations, gels, pessaries and lotions.

The conventional route for herbalists in Britain is to train for four years with the School of Phytotherapy in East Sussex, leading to membership of the National Institute of Medical Herbalists.

Rosalind also went on to train with Dr Daniel Penoël, a French doctor and expert in aromatic medicine. With him she now runs specialist aromatic medicine training courses for qualified herbalists, naturopaths and doctors . . . as well as organising her own busy practices.

Some patients come to her as a first port of call for diagnosis, as well as treatment, while others may have already had their problem diagnosed by a GP, but have opted to tackle it with herbal therapy. The process works both ways - there are often cases where the herbalist will advise patients to see their GP.

A first consultation with a herbalist takes up to an hour, and will include taking a full medical history and carrying out a physical examination, if necessary. A vital skill for any practitioner is building the patient's confidence in the treatment, because a favourable expectation of the outcome - the placebo effect - is generally recognised as an important factor in the healing process. But does it play more of a part in herbal therapy than in conventional medicine?

Far from it, says Rosalind Blackwell. "I think herbal medicine is one of the easiest systems of medicine to rationalise because we know that the plants have certain biological effects on the tissues, organs and systems. We know that they contain various chemicals, that they have molecules in them that work on a pharmacological level, so we know that you are going to get certain effects if you take them.

"A lot of people will be helped to an extent by whatever they take. There is always a certain placebo effect in any sort of treatment because you always have expectations for it and you feel you are doing something positive to help yourself.

"It really amounts to a positive attitude. It's just a little helpful extra, but the treatment is certainly not placebo orientated.

"You can give people herbal treatment when they're not really expecting anything at all. They might even have been coerced into it by somebody in the family and you can still get excellent results."

The way that herbalists use herbs is very different from the simpler approach of self-treatment. Herbalists are knowledgeable about a huge range of herbs, many of which have overlapping effects, and they all tend to have their favourites. Some, like Rosalind Blackwell, use peppermint quite a lot, others may use it less.

They also tend to use plant extracts in combination rather than singly, so they would be unlikely to give peppermint on its own. More typical would be the giving of peppermint in combination with up to six herbs, the choice of which may vary according to the particular needs of each patient.

Finally, in herbalism treatment of symptoms is only part of the picture. Practitioners will also encourage changes in lifestyle and nutrition, and will look at emotional, as well as physical, problems.

To be fair to National Health Service doctors, many of them also adopt as much of an holistic approach to health care as their workload allows, but herbalists, who are after all charging a fee for treatment, usually have far more scope to do so because they have the time to go into each patient's case in depth.

"We have a naturopathic view of the systems of the body," says Rosalind Blackwell. "The naturopathic or holistic view is one that takes into account everything; we look to see the causes of the problem, not just the symptoms.

"So it would be bad practice for a herbal practitioner to treat somebody just with peppermint for dyspepsia and not investigate underlying causes because it may be that there is a serious problem, or a lot of tension in their lives or that they are eating really badly, so you would have to adjust their diet and you might suggest ways of relaxation and other things as well.

"It is important to eliminate a serious cause of the symptoms, but it is just as bad to treat symptomatically with herbs as it is with orthodox medicine. Of course the difference is that mostly the herbs we use are non-toxic and not going to have the side effects that drugs can have."

The risk of side effects from taking peppermint is small, but there are limits on daily intake and there are circumstances in which it should be avoided altogether - see the section on Safety and Toxicity in Chapter 3.

Rosalind Blackwell does not prescribe oil of peppermint for more than a month at a time without allowing a break from it. Peppermint tea is a pleasant digestive aid, but again she recommends moderation if you use it fairly regularly . . . a couple of cups in a day, although not every day, is fine, but not four or five.

She prescribes peppermint both as a tincture and as an oil to use in a variety of ways, as part of a topical massage formula, for inhaling or sometimes to take internally, in which case she would usually add 1 drop to a formula in a capsule or an emulsion for a single dose.

How a herbalist prescribes peppermint

"I would use tincture of peppermint as part of a formula quite often in the case of **colds**, **catarrh**, **flatulence**, **dyspepsia**, **colicky pain**, the sort of things that it's classically known for, but I do use essential oil of peppermint quite a lot as well . . . if I wanted a stronger effect I would use the oil.

"If I were treating babies or children, for instance, I wouldn't use the essential oil, but would use the whole plant extract. The whole plant is a gentler, more dilute form and you can use it in a higher dosage.

"Oil of peppermint could certainly form part of a topical application for **arthritis** because it does have analgesic effects in the essential oil. As an internal treatment it could be very useful, always combined with other botanicals, because of its detoxifying effects on the liver and bowel. It is vital to treat the liver and bowel in both osteo and rheumatoid arthritis. It also has an invigorating effect. Well-being generally could certainly be improved with peppermint because it is a tonic.

"Peppermint is very good for people who are rather what is called asthenic, suffering from weakness and debility, maybe as a constitutional thing, or part of post-illness, so in **convalescence** it's a very good nerve tonic to use."

Peppermint oil often forms part of the treatment for **liver disorders**. It stimulates and increases the production of bile, a secretion of the liver which aids digestion and bowel function.

"It has an excellent tonic effect after infections to stimulate the liver and is also used for chronic hepatitis. It is good for the liver cells. I've been treating someone using peppermint who has had a very bad liver condition. He is at the one extreme of liver disorders with quite a serious problem.

"Orthodox medicine couldn't offer anything except a low-fat diet and plenty of rest, but there are a number of very good plant remedies - peppermint isn't the only one - for treating the liver. At the other end of the spectrum, an awful lot of people are not very well just because of the toxic input through daily life from all sorts of sources. They haven't got liver disease, they have just got sluggish systems - they may have got constipation due to a sluggish liver. Peppermint is absolutely ideal for that. Herbalists do pay a great deal of attention to the function of the liver because it is involved in so many different processes in the body."

Peppermint's anaesthetic effect on the stomach helps allay the nausea in **morning sickness in pregnancy**.

"I wouldn't prescribe essential oil of peppermint in pregnancy to take internally. I'd use the whole plant in a tea or tincture. It would be OK to use essential oils externally in small amounts, but it's something you do under guidance of a herbalist.

"You wouldn't use much peppermint oil externally if pregnant, but if I had a pregnant woman, as I did recently with a sinus infection, I would make up some essential oil to apply externally to the sinus area and I would quite happily put 1 drop of peppermint or spearmint oil in the formula; that wouldn't worry me at all, just for a week or so. You could certainly use the tea internally in pregnancy within reasonable limits."

Peppermint is a decongestant of the **prostate**, the gland surrounding the male urethra at its junction with the bladder, and can be helpful in treating **benign enlargement**, especially in the early stages. **Prostatitis** is an inflamed swollen prostate usually resulting from infection. Peppermint oil's antiseptic, detoxifying properties make it an appropriate treatment in both conditions, which have a broad range of underlying causes, in combination with other herbal extracts.

"For prostate problems you would need peppermint oil in quite high concentrations. If it becomes a real nuisance then the answer is surgery, either to shave it down a bit or remove portions of it. Certainly in the early stages it is worth using peppermint."

In benign enlargement, peppermint does not reduce the enlargement but improves general local conditions, so treatment can help avoid the need for surgery, at least for many years.

"Peppermint has hormone-like properties and it helps to regulate the cycle of the ovaries, so it can be used in **period problems**. That would be the essential oil. As a professional, if you were treating period problems you would invariably be using it in a formula because you would be using things that are both oestrogen-like and progesterone-like in different parts of the cycle. But peppermint could form part of that treatment certainly.

Menstrual problems can provoke an irritable bowel, causing painful spasms, and Rosalind would always use peppermint oil in a formula in IBS, usually with a demulcent herb like marshmallow or slippery elm and sometimes with valerian if there is a lot of stress.

"It's extremely active against **cold sores** and **shingles**, which are both caused by herpes viruses, and I use peppermint externally extensively in a formula with the herbs ravensara and callophylum in these conditions.

"In **sciatica** I would use peppermint as a massage oil to give pain relief. It is very good in a formula; usually lavender and rosemary go well."

Two case histories

A man in his 30s had a serious problem with liver function. He was very jaundiced with skin that itched so much that it disturbed his sleep. He had bleeding gums, was nauseous after food (especially if fatty), complained of aching, had indigestion and had lost weight.

The problem had been a recurrent one since his teens and he had had a liver biopsy three years before. The mainstay of orthodox treatment was diet and rest, although he also had drugs, which seemed not to help. His urine was dark and stools pale, a common feature where there is obstruction of the bile ducts. Tests also showed an abnormality of bile salts (they help digest fat) in his urine. His blood pressure was low. His diet needed no adjustment, being already low in fat, high in fibre and alcohol-free.

The initial prescription, for three weeks, was one formula combining peppermint (some of it being essential oil) and milk thistle, plus a digestive aid, which contained charcoal, slippery elm and other extracts.

Three weeks later there was a significant improvement, although still bile salts in the urine. The patient was given a new prescription of milk thistle, meadowsweet and marshmallow - peppermint was allowed a three-week break.

A further three weeks saw more improvement, including weight gain, and normal blood pressure. Skin itching was much better, although digestion was still not right. The prescription this time again included peppermint tincture and essential oil, as well as milk thistle, dandelion root and essence of lemon.

The next visit was the final one, as the patient was back to normal weight, his jaundice had cleared and he was thoroughly well.

A woman in her 60s reported severe pains in the left side of the head (extending down whole of the left side). She had perpetual nausea and had been vomiting. Several sessions with an acupuncturist had already helped before she consulted the medical herbalist.

The pain was from migraine due to gall bladder problems, of which the patient had a history, but gallstones had not been shown in tests. The gall bladder was, however, found to be extremely tender after palpitation. Bowel action was also erratic.

On this first visit the patient was given a head and neck massage with essential oils of lavender and peppermint dotted neat on the temples and the base of the skull. There was also a prescription of oil of peppermint; 2 drops per dose, three doses a day, to be reduced to twice daily as symptoms subsided.

After three weeks the headaches had diminished considerably and a new prescription, which included a number of extracts, among them peppermint and feverfew, was given. Returning three weeks later the patient reported feeling well, with her digestion improved, headaches gone and bowel function normal.

How an aromatherapist uses peppermint

Katrina Roberts has been practising as an aromatherapist for four years. Massage is the basis of most of the aromatherapy treatment she gives, and for that oil of peppermint has various applications, sometimes on its own, but more frequently in a mix with other oils.

In Katrina's experience people often have aromatherapy as an adjunct to other forms of treatment, perhaps on the recommendation of GPs or other alternative practitioners.

"A lot of women who are having hormone replacement therapy come to me on the recommendation of their GP for aromatherapy as relaxation. If they were suffering from **headaches** I might use peppermint. I would massage it into the whole of the back of the neck, up the neck and shoulder muscles where tension creates a lot of the pain, and possibly also into the temples and the forehead. I'm always careful with peppermint because it can be irritating if you use it on the skin. The only other time I would use peppermint on the face is for **sinus problems**.

"I do quite a lot of **massage** on men, and for that peppermint is one of the most frequently-used oils because it's quite a refreshing, 'masculine' aroma, whereas a lot of the other oils are quite floral. Men don't want to go back to the office after a massage at lunchtime and have people comment on how fragrant they are!

"Peppermint is very good as a **pre-sports rub** to prewarm the muscles. I would use it with rosemary to speed up the circulation, so that the muscles receive fresh supplies of blood and oxygen. They then do a better job and it lessens the tendency to cramp.

"What happens when you are massaging is that you are actually helping to bring extra blood supplies to the surface, making it easier for the oil to be absorbed, and all the squeezing and releasing of tissues stimulates the blood stream to carry the oils around the body.

"As an **after-sports treatment** I often use peppermint with lavender and rosemary. If someone has torn a muscle, for instance, I put on an ice-pack, like a bag of frozen peas wrapped in a tea towel (so it isn't in direct contact with the skin) for 10-15 minutes. Then they soak in a bath with a few drops of thyme and rosemary before I massage peppermint and lavender into the affected area. After that I apply a warm compress.

"As a compress I use what is called an aromaplasm. It is made from linseed oil, sesame and sunflower seeds, bran and all sorts of whole grains, which are ground down and made into a paste. I warm it up, spread it over the area and leave it on until it has cooled right down.

"A number of people complain of **irritable bowel syndrome**. A lot of it is stress causing the whole body to malfunction and the stomach and intestines are one of the first areas to be hit by the tension. I often find that the solar plexus (a network of nerves, veins and lymphatic vessels adjacent to the stomach) feels tense and hard like a tight ball, and by massaging in an anti-clockwise direction you can have an effect on the whole body.

"I have used peppermint with marjoram in a blend for bad **constipation**, in which case I might massage the stomach area. The actual movement on that area seems to help stimulate the bowel.

"I have treated people who have goosebumps, little areas of dry skin, a rough prickly surface on the top of thighs and arms which is a sign of poor **circulation**. It's a cosmetic thing, but it can be a sign that the circulatory system internally isn't functioning properly. Poor circulation means that the body is not being detoxified as well as it could be. Peppermint can help detoxify the system by speeding up the circulation and getting the toxins released more efficiently from the tissues. I might use it in conjunction with geranium which will have a diuretic effect and helps to flush the toxins out of the system. Also related to circulation, I have used peppermint as a foot massage, mainly for **chilblains**. The massage itself will improve the circulation, as well as the actual oil."

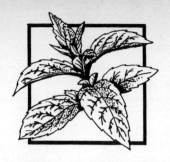

CHAPTER EIGHT

Commercial developments with peppermint

The relationship between traditional herbal remedies and modern drugs has always been closer than the natural-versus-synthetic stereotypes would suggest. Ingredients lists of many familiar, long-established medicines, generally thought of as pharmaceutical products, include plant material or single plant extracts. Other drugs, although synthetic, are made from an original formula based on the chemical structure of a plant substance.

Plant remedies such as peppermint have in recent years experienced a renaissance in mainstream popular medicine. It has become the norm for pharmacies and supermarkets, as well as health food shops which have always specialised in natural medicines, to sell herbal products for self treatment. This has come about partly from specialist herbal medicine manufacturers widening their market, but also from a growing interest among pharmaceutical companies in botanical medicine.

Peppermint is a plant substance whose pharmacological properties have been recognised by the pharmaceutical industry and there are on the market two products made from peppermint oil and officially licensed as medicines. They are available to buy over-the-counter, but because they are promoted to doctors, advertising to the general public is not permitted and virtually all sales are through prescriptions (for irritable bowel).

Most peppermint remedies sold over-the-counter in health food shops and chemists are officially categorised as food supplements, rather than medicines. This means that although they have to meet safety criteria, the manufacturers are not permitted to make any medicinal claims or indicate the products' medicinal uses on the packaging.

There are many herbal products which come into this quasi-medicinal category in Britain . . . they come in medicinal forms, capsules, tablets, mixtures and so on, they are presented and packaged as medicines, but officially they are not considered to have medicinal uses.

This state of affairs does not apply universally to plant medicines on sale in Britain, many of which are licensed by the Department of Health as medicines and are permitted to make claims for certain specified conditions. They are usually either products which have been on the market for decades, so have medicinal licences by virtue of long-established use, or are made by pharmaceutical companies because the enormous costs involved in obtaining medicinal licences for new products are often a deterrent for small, specialist herbal medicine manufacturers.

Licensing systems for medicines vary from country to country. In Denmark, which is where one of the best-known brands of over-the-counter peppermint remedies (Obbekjaers) is made, there is a two-tier system enabling natural products to obtain a simplified licence (there has been some discussion of introducing a similar system in the UK). Manufacturers, who must demonstrate the product's safety, are permitted to make limited medicinal claims in self-limiting ailments, but do not need to produce the amount of scientific evidence of efficacy that would be required for medicines used in more serious conditions.

Obbekjaers peppermint oil is promoted as an oral medication for the treatment of irritable bowel, heartburn, restless legs and night cramps and as a topical rub for muscular aches and pains.

The origins of Obbekjaers (pronounced Obbercares), the best-known brand of peppermint oil sold in British health food shops, is a colourful story, typical of herbal medicine and involving one individual's personal enthusiasm being transformed into a sizeable business.

Erhardt Obbekjaer, who originally produced the formulation which developed into the products which are now sold around Europe, the United States and Canada, lived most of his life in provincial Denmark. The success of Obbekjaers oil of peppermint brought a measure of fame for him personally and his name, which would have probably seemed incredible to him when he retired after nearly 40 years of service as the manager of a potato flour mill in Oelsted, a village in northern Denmark.

His involvement in commercial production of oil of peppermint came only as a belated second career when he was in his 70s. But his fascination with herbs went back to his youth, to when he was training in agriculture and had spent several years working on farms. He went on to study agronomy at the Royal Veterinary and Agricultural College in Copenhagen, followed by a course in bacteriology. Subsequently he did various jobs involved in food technology and the science of crop production and at one time was running his own agricultural laboratory.

He had some professional experience of plant oils during his working life, but it was only after retirement and as a result of personal circumstances that he became so enthusiastic about peppermint. In 1968, at the age of 72, he had a car accident, which caused 11 fractures and concussion, and he was in hospital for several months. He then had several strokes and suffered memory loss which left him feeling badly depressed.

But "Old Obbekjaer", as his friends affectionately knew
him, had plenty of spirit and was determined to try anything to improve his health. The choice of peppermint as a
possible tonic was not an entirely random one. Erhardt
was familiar with its traditional medicinal use, but when
he added a drop of peppermint oil one evening to his
habitual glass of home-made wine it was more in the spirit of "even if it doesn't do any good, it can't do any harm"
than conviction.

However, Erhardt did enjoy dramatically improved
health, and he became convinced that this was due to his
regular doses of peppermint. Not only did he continue to
take peppermint daily, but he also gave it to friends and
neighbours, although he did switch from adding it to
wine to mixing it with a type of sugar, dextrose. As the
dextrose was quickly absorbed into the bloodstream, he
reasoned, it would also speed up peppermint's assimila-
tion.

Relief from digestive complaints, cramp, varicose veins
and migraine was reported. Some people even claimed
that their eyesight was improved and that rheumatic and
arthritic pain was alleviated.

After the appearance of a newspaper article, Erhardt
soon found himself inundated with requests for his mixture and had a growing mail order business on his hands.
Eventually he sold the production and sales rights to a
health food company. Obbekjaers products have been
sold in the UK since the late '70s. Advertising and promo-
tion of the brand has generated newspaper and magazine
coverage fostering a renewed popular interest in peppermint as a remedy for self-treatment.

Also towards the end of the '70s - in 1979 - the results of
a small study carried out among gastroenterological
patients demonstrating the effectiveness of oil of peppermint in the treatment of irritable bowel syndrome
appeared in the pages of the *British Medical Journal*[48]. It

was couched in the usual, dry scientific language . . . and as medical trials go it was not going to set the world ablaze. Peppermint was a useful treatment, not a cure-all, although significantly beneficial in a common, albeit not a life-threatening complaint in one of the less glamorous areas of medicine. Hardly the stuff of which headlines are made, or from which human interest stories are spun. Yet behind the gravitas of the medical journal hangs quite a tale.

Brian Evans was a young hospital pharmacist at the University Hospital of Wales at Heath Park, Cardiff, in the early '70s wanting to take a postgraduate degree. As is fairly routine in these matters he approached a lecturer at the University College in Cardiff, of which he was a graduate and where he planned to take his Masters, asking what topics would be available for research. One of them was to further explore a scientific principle, the Ferguson principle, named after a chemist who back in the 1930s had studied various chemical compounds which, although chemically unrelated (they were composed of molecules of totally different structure), all had a similar pharmacological action. Ferguson had concluded that this action was determined by a physical feature - their degree of solubility in water.

Brian Evans had been interested in this principle since his undergraduate days, but it was also his passion for gardening and his love of aromatic herbs that determined his choice of thesis, studying Ferguson's principle in relation to plant extracts, in particular volatile oils, one of which was menthol from peppermint. Historical uses of herbs were pointers to various lines of research that might be fruitful; their traditional use as stomachic remedies, for instance, prompted tests on how they affected smooth muscle contraction.

The finding, among many others, that they all had a soothing action on smooth muscle contraction[59], helped prove Brian Evans's point, but it was rather the result he had expected, so it was not earth-shattering. That would have been as far as it went, he says, had it not been for conversations with a hospital gastroenterologist colleague, then Dr, now Professor, John Rhodes, about the large numbers of sufferers with irritable bowel and other smooth muscle-related conditions at outpatients' clinics, and the limited range of drugs suitable for treatment.

The plant extracts that Brian Evans had been studying seemed to offer a possible new type of medication; the next stage was to decide which one to develop into a formula suitable for administering to patients. Oil of peppermint was chosen mainly because menthol was one of the most effective of all the oils in relaxing muscle contraction; it was also widely used in the UK in confectionery and toothpastes, so was a familiar substance. Its comparative safety as a drug was also a plus point; the amount that Evans and Rhodes planned to use was well within the World Health Organisation's acceptable daily intake level. It was, and still is, monographed in the *British Pharmacopoeia*, a standard reference book on drugs.

They chose oil of peppermint in its whole form, rather than an extract of its most active ingredient, menthol, because there was not much information available on acceptable intakes of menthol, leaving more of a question mark over its safety. More positively, they wondered whether the other components in the oil might work synergistically with the menthol . . . in other words, that the whole might be more effective than the sum of its separate parts.

Early research among patients, indicating that it was in irritable bowel syndrome that the treatment was most effective, led to several more years of study. Brian Evans, who had along the way converted his Masters degree into a doctorate, spent much of his spare time manufacturing peppermint capsules, Heath Robinson-style, for clinical trials and subsequently to supply doctors who contacted him after reading the initial report of his work in the *British Medical Journal* in 1979.

Eventually, unable to meet the demand, he offered the formula to a pharmaceutical company, Tillots Laboratories, who reformulated it and launched a product called Colpermin in the early 1980s. Colpermin, now marketed by a company called Farmitalia, and a second product, Mintec, are today widely prescribed by gastroenterologists and GPs treating irritable bowel syndrome.

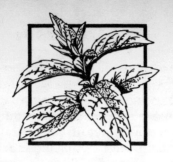

CHAPTER NINE

Peppermint cultivated

Peppermint's place in the plant kingdom

The plant kingdom is like a sprawling tribe of incredibly diverse family groups, who can nevertheless claim that somewhere, way back in the past, they share a common descent.

The kingdom is split into divisions (phylums), which in turn break down into classes, orders and then different families; the families are then divided into genera (genus is the singular) and the genera into different species.

Right at the end of this vast tribal tree are further groups, sub-species, varieties and forms, identifying subtle variations within each species.

How does peppermint fit into this scheme of things? Is it a family, is it a genus, or is it a variety?

Peppermint is a species, one of many in the mint or Mentha genus. This genus is part of the Labiatae family, which contains around 3,000 plants and falls within the flowering plant division of the plant kingdom.

Tradition has it that peppermint (*Mentha x piperita L.*)*

---

* The x in the description denotes a hybrid. L refers to Linnaeus, the Swedish botanist who gave the Latin name.

was originally a hybrid (a cross breed) between two other species of mint, spearmint (*Mentha viridis or Mentha spicata*) and water mint (*Mentha aquatica*), although there has never been universal agreement on the point. Within the peppermint species there are numerous varieties and forms, but two main ones: white peppermint (*Mentha piperita var officinalis*) and black peppermint (*Mentha piperita var vulgaris*)*. The black is a hardier plant, with higher yields of oil, while the oil from white peppermint is said to be superior.

In the Mentha genus generally, the huge range of species and varieties and the fact that some have several vernacular names, and even more than one Latin name, makes identification and classification an ever-evolving discipline.

For the amateur gardener, the array of mints can be bewildering. In all there are more than 2,000 different names for mints[18] and around 30 - even more according to some sources - are recognised as true species. One of the most authoritative classifications in this country has been done at Rosemary Titterington's Iden Croft Herb Garden at Staplehurst in Kent, where she has a range of around 30 distinct species and varieties of mints, including the black and the white peppermint. Growers and experts were invited to the nursery during the summer of 1991 to a special open day to inspect and identify various mint plants, all grown in similar pots and composts. As part of the exercise, participants were asked to give what they considered to be the correct Latin name for each species, reaching more or less a consensus.

Like most plants in the Labiatae family, which includes basil, rosemary, oregano, lavender, marjoram, lemon balm, sage and thyme, mints produce aromatic (essential) oils from their leaves and stems.

* There are various Latin names for them.

The best-known medicinally-active ingredient found in the oil of most types of mint is menthol. Peppermint has one of the highest contents of menthol among the mints, but higher still is *Mentha arvensis*, field or corn mint as it is called. It is commonly referred to as Japanese mint, or Japanese peppermint, but although similar to *piperita*, it is a different species. *Mentha arvensis* is a hardy, robust plant which reaches 80cm in height. It has a purple stem and dark green leaves.

Peppermint in the garden

An English Tourist Board signpost on the main Newbury to Andover road at Woolton Hill in Hampshire directs visitors down leafy lanes to Hollington Herb Garden, another fine example of that quintessentially English establishment, the specialist herb nursery.

Set in a walled garden, it's a restful stopover for the passing motorist, a wonderland for the serious gardener, and a flourishing illustration of the fascinating variety to be found among common herbs like mint.

There are nurseries like Hollington and Rosemary Titterington's Iden Croft Herb Garden all over the country, and it is to such establishments that the would-be peppermint cultivator should make tracks . . . certainly to find plants and seek advice, but also for the opportunity to see a range of mints in one place and to compare their appearance and smell. Just rub a few leaves of several types of mint and you will discover their particular fragrances are often quite distinct.

Peppermint has pinky, lilac flowers and its broad leaves are light green on the white variety and darker on the black peppermint. It has a pungent, sweet aroma and taste. It looks similar to spearmint, although its leaves are less wrinkled.

Spearmint is the species most commonly grown in gardens because of its culinary suitability, and is probably the most familiar in appearance, but some other species bear little resemblance to it at all. Corsican mint, for instance, has tiny blue flowers and its leaves are minute. There are variegated forms of mints, others have almost purple leaves, there is *Mentha crispa* or curly mint which, as its name suggests, has crinkly leaves, some types have grey foliage, while others such as apple mint have hairy leaves and stems.

The shape and arrangement of the leaves vary too. Some are long and thin, others are round, certain types sprout from a single stem like Bowles mint and lemon mint, while ginger mint, for instance, has lots of smaller stems branching off. Flowers come in varying shades of blue, pink and purple.

Besides the typical culinary patch of spearmint, other types of mint are usually grown purely ornamentally, says Judith Hopkinson of Hollington Nurseries, although eau-de-cologne, which is a close relation of peppermint and is, to most noses, the most sweet-smelling of the mints, adds a fresh fragrance to the home-grown pot pourri bowl. Other mints recommended for the cooking pot from the Iden Croft herb collection include Moroccan mint (*Mentha spicata* "Moroccan") and variegated apple mint (*Mentha suaveolens variegata*).

Herb enthusiasts often cultivate peppermint simply out of a spirit of acquisition. Having caught the herb-growing bug, they gather as many mint species and varieties as they can, and peppermint is an addition to the collection.

But peppermint can earn a place in a practical garden, especially one whose owners enjoy herb tea. It is also useful planted near roses because its essential oil helps keep aphids at bay.

Propagation

Serious gardeners and nursery growers cultivate new

mint plants by propagation - growing from parent stock - rather than from seed because of mint's tendency to cross-pollinate and produce hybrids.

The first opportunity to take cuttings from a pepper-mint plant is April time. Take around 2 or 3 inches from a sturdy, low-growing stem, remove the lower leaves, dip in water and then some hormone rooting powder, and plant in rooting compost. Leave in a warm, moist greenhouse atmosphere for two or three weeks before transferring into larger pots and cutting back to about 1 inch to encourage bushy growth.

Rust

All mints are prone to the ravages of rust, a parasitic fun-gus whose spores lurk in the soil latching on to the leaves and stem as the plant grows. The rust cannot be seen until it has got a hold on a plant, by which time it will have produced unsightly red patches over the leaves and stem, will have killed off some of the growth and weakened the plant.

There is no certain cure for rust although, if you are growing peppermint as an ornamental plant, a dose of fungicide may be moderately effective. It's not advisable, though, to use such treatment if you are going to be mak-ing tea from the leaves. All you can do is to dig up and burn badly affected plants and start again with a fresh supply. A precautionary measure is to cut off all old shoots at the end of the growing season.

Whether peppermint is grown in a pot, a window-box or in a garden bed, it is quite adaptable; it will take fairly heavy shade for a good part of the day and is one of the few herbs that will grow in total shade, although commer-cially it is usually grown under the full glare of the sun. It prefers a rich, loam or loam-clay soil, rich in humus, and needs plenty of water.

Feeding

In theory peppermint will go on growing year in, year out, but if you have a "working" plant, being cropped regularly, it will probably have a limited lifetime.

Certainly, to produce regular large crops of leaves in a summer, the plant will need feeding with a liquid feed every two weeks.

May or June is the time to take the first crop from an established plant. If you leave cropping too long, the leaves will lose some of their flavour since exposure to the sun causes some of the plant's essential oils to evaporate, although sun increases its menthol content.

After a six to eight weeks' rest, the plant should give a second crop, and a healthy plant may even grow back to produce a third harvest at the end of the summer. Be thorough each time you harvest and take off most of the leaves - they will soon start to grow back. In between the main croppings you can also take small quantities for day-to-day use, but once the plant's full bloom is finished the leaves will be past their best.

The best time of day to harvest is in the morning when it is already warm enough for the dew to have cleared, but before the sun is really hot.

Growing indoors

Peppermint can be grown indoors to provide fresh herbs through the winter. Ideally keep half-a-dozen pots or so on the go, so that each one only needs to spend a few weeks indoors. Thus you have two inside, at any one time, one supplying fresh peppermint, the other coming on to replace it after about a month, and the others resting in the open air.

Preserving peppermint

The leaves are best dried in thin layers on racks, trays or

flat cardboard boxes covered with cheese cloth or kitchen paper to keep off the dust. Twenty-four hours in somewhere like an airing cupboard, or a darkened greenhouse where there is a gentle heat, between 70°F (21°C) and 90°F and (32°C) should leave the peppermint brittle and dry, but not blackened. The ideal containers for storing dried herbs are dark-glass bottles, kept in a cool place.

For speed and simplicity nothing beats freezing peppermint, including whole stems, and it is also the most efficient way of preserving the essential oils of the herb. Once defrosted the leaves are soggy, but fine for making tea.

Flavouring with peppermint

Although not the most usual culinary herb, the taste of peppermint does lend itself to some foods, especially fruits. Arabella Boxer and Philippa Back's *The Herb Book* suggests the addition of peppermint to fruit juices and fruit salads, and sprinkling it on split pea soup, carrots and courgettes. A few chopped peppermint leaves make a cup of hot chocolate or cocoa a little more interesting, and they can also be added to regular black tea.

(See the Useful addresses section for details of specialist herb nurseries.)

Peppermint on the farm

Mentha piperita is now grown around the world, in subtropical as well as temperate climes; the USA is the main supplier. *Mentha arvensis*, known as Japanese mint or Japanese peppermint, is also grown extensively, but only a small amount comes from Japan, the major sources being China and Brazil. Although it has a higher menthol content, it is considered to have an inferior aroma and flavour.

Mentha piperita has been an important crop in the USA since the last century, but during the 1980s became particularly lucrative for farmers, particularly in Ohio, Oregon and Washington State, which are still among the main growing areas. An average acreage on a farm would be a total of around 600-700 and in 1992 total yield was expected to be around 6 million lbs of peppermint.

New plants are grown from cuttings and nurtured in nursery conditions, before being thinned and then planted out in the fields using fairly basic technology. A lorry with two ploughshare-type devices fitted to the front digs two trenches ready for the peppermint plants, which are being sorted by farmhands on the back of the lorry, to be dropped in by two conveyor belts.

Another reversed ploughshare attached to the back of the lorry covers the plants with earth, then all they need is plenty of water - and sometimes strictly controlled sprays of herbicide - for them to grow. Rust, the plague of British mints, has been bred out of the US stock, although it is sometimes assaulted by a condition called wilt which can reduce the yield. Peppermint is pretty hardy stuff, though, and once planted out on a US farm will, as long as it gets plenty of water, produce a crop for two or three, even as many as seven, seasons.

Planting of new plants is in March and April, while harvesting, by means of a machine taking the tops off all the plants, including the flowers, starts at the earliest in July and continues through August and September. Cropping is done when the leaves are at their greenest and lushest.

In sub-tropical climates and the foothills of India the growth is quicker, with the plant covering the entire field after the rains; two or three crops may be taken in a season.

Climate does affect the chemical make-up of the oil. To produce a high menthol content, the peppermint needs to have around 14 hours of daylight and plenty of sun during harvest time because in cloudy weather some of the menthol converts into menthone[23].

Grown domestically, it makes no odds whether a peppermint plant has a slightly reduced proportion of menthol, and in fact a high menthol content does not necessarily improve the taste. In the commercial world, though, where menthol content is an important factor in marketing the oil, and peppermint is being grown in huge quantities, it is critical.

Distillation to remove the plants' oil content is done virtually immediately on the farm, the peppermint being put into a metal container and heated with steam until the oil is forced out. It is then condensed and put into drums, then is ready to be supplied to oil processors, who may blend the piperita with oil from other areas, or with arvensis, or add extra menthol, producing a variety of products to suit different markets.

Around 910 tonnes of peppermint oil is imported annually into the UK, where its greatest use is in flavouring toothpaste. It also goes into confectionery, toiletries, drinks, medicines and aromatherapy oils. Interestingly, there is limited demand for synthetic peppermint - most manufacturers prefer the real thing.

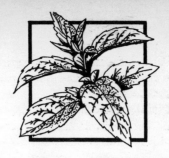

Useful addresses

One of the best-known brands of peppermint oil products available in health food shops and chemists is Obbekjaers. The range includes capsules, tablets, fibre tablets, powder and dropper bottles of oil, and is available in the UK through:

Bennett Natural Products
Wheelton
Chorley
Lancashire PR6 8EP

0245 831520

Other brands include:

Healthilife Ltd (tablets)
Charleston House
Otley Road
Baildon
Shipley
West Yorkshire BD17 7JS

0274 595021/5

Power Health Products Ltd (capsules, bottled oil, cream)
10 Central Avenue
Airfield Estate
Pocklington
York YO4 2NR

0759 302734

Brands available on NHS prescription and over the counter from chemists are:

Colpermin

Farmitalia Carlo Erba Ltd
Italia House
23 Grosvenor Road
St Albans
Hertfordshire AL1 3AW

0727 40041

Mintec

Novex Pharma Ltd
Innovex House
309 Reading Road
Henley-on-Thames
Oxfordshire RG9 1EL

0491 578171

Various herbal medicines contain peppermint as part of their formulation. One of the best-known herbal cold treatments is Elderflowers with Peppermint and Composition Essence.

Potter's (Herbal Supplies) Ltd
Leyland Mill Lane
Wigan
Lancashire WN1 2SB

0942 34761

There are many aromatherapy oil suppliers whose ranges include peppermint. This is far from a comprehensive round-up, but among leading brands are:

Gerard House Ltd
3 Wickham Road
Boscombe
Bournemouth
Dorset BH7 6JX

0202 434116

Natural by Nature Oils Ltd
27 Vivian Avenue
Hendon Central
London NW4 3UX

081-202 5718

Nelson & Russell Aromatherapy
5 Endeavour Way
Wimbledon
London SW19 9UH

081-946 8527

Tisserand Aromatherapy
Aromatherapy Products Ltd
Unit W3
The Knoll Business Centre
Old Shoreham Road
Hove
Sussex BN3 7GS

0273 412139

Numerous brands of peppermint tea are now available in health food shops and chemists. They include Heath & Heather, London Herb and Spice Company, Jill Davies, Pompadour, and Cotswold Health Products.

Other useful addresses

British Digestive Foundation
7 Chandos Street
London W1A 2LN

For information send SAE.

For a list of medical herbalists and aromatherapists write (with SAE) to:

National Institute of Medical Herbalists
9 Palace Gate
Exeter EX1 1JA

International Federation of Aromatherapists
Department of Continuing Education
Royal Masonic Hospital
Ravenscourt Park
London W6 0TN

or

The Association of Tisserand Aromatherapists
PO Box 746
Hove BN3 3XA

For information about specialist herb nurseries write
(with SAE) to:

British Herb Trade Association
Agriculture House
Knightsbridge
London SW1X 7NJ

or

The Herb Society
PO Box 599
London SW11 4RW

(for professionals and amateur enthusiasts. The Herb
Society publishes the journal *Herbs*, formerly *The Herbal
Review*)

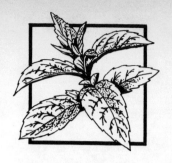

Sources

1. *Healing Herbs of the Bible*, Harrison (E. J. Brill, 1966)

2. *Obbekjaer*, Foged (Denmark, 1978), pp 60-72

3. *Nature's Pharmacy*, Stockwell (Century, 1988), p 56

4. *Green Pharmacy*, Griggs (Hale, 1981), pp 10, 13, 271-2

5. *Chinese Materia Medica*, Stuart (American Presbyterian Press, 1911)

6. *Chinese Herbal Medicine*, Reid (CFW Publications, 1987), p 10

7. *Secrets of the Chinese Herbalists*, Lucas (Thorsons, 1978), p 19

8. *The Art of Aromatherapy*, Tisserand (C. W. Daniel, 1979), pp 26, 101, 266-270

9. Pliny's *Natural History* (vols X1X and XX) (Heinemann/Harvard University Press)

10. *Herbs* (Herb Society journal), autumn/winter 1991, pp 12-14

11. *Herbs*, autumn/winter 1990, pp 2-4

12. *A Modern Herbal*, Mrs M. Grieve (Penguin, 1980),pp 532-546

13. *Leaves from Gerard's Herball*, arrgd by Woodward (facsimile ed, Thorsons, 1972)

14. *Culpeper's Complete Herbal* (Omega Books, 1985), pp 190-192

15. *Lark Rise to Candleford*, Thompson (Penguin), p 115

16. *The Story of Lavender*, Festing (Heritage in Sutton Leisure), pp 8, 49, 54, 62, 65, 67, 74, 99

17. John Parkinson, *Theatrum Botanicum*, 1640

18. *Peppermint*, Foster (American Botanical Council leaflet)

19. *Ethnobotany of the Menomini Indians*, Smith (Bulletin of the Public Museum of Milwaukee, 1923), p 39

20. *Meals Medicinal*, Dr W. T. Fernie (1905)

21. *Volatile Oils*, Alfred Hall

22. *The Practice of Aromatherapy*, Valnet (C. W. Daniel, 1980), pp 33-34, 69, 172-174

23. *The Medicinal Plant Industry*, Wijesekera (CRC Press, 1991), pp 45, 56-57

24. Harries et al, *British Journal of Clinical Pharmacology*, 1978; 2: p 171

25. Sigmund and McNally, *Gastroenterology*, 1969; 56: p 13

26. Proposal for a European Monography on the medicinal use of peppermint oil by the European Scientific Cooperative for Phytotherapy (version 7, 1992)

27. *The A-Z of Modern Herbalism*, Mills, (Thorsons, 1989) pp 79, 165-166

28. *The International Journal of Aromatherapy*, Spring 1992; volume 4: No 1, pp 20-25

29. *The Energetics of Western Herbs*, Holmes (Artemis Press), pp 107-109

30. Taddei et al, *Fitoterapia*. 1988 ;59: pp 463-468

31. Schafer et al, *Journal of General Physiology* 1986; 88: pp 757-776

32. *Thorsons Guide to Medical Herbalism*, Hoffmann (1991), pp 27-28

33. Cohen and Dressler, *Respiration*, 1982; 43: pp 285-293

34. Eccles et al, *Journal of Pharmacy and Pharmacology*, 1990; 42: pp 652-654

35. Eccles and Jones, *Journal of Laryngology and Otology*, 1983; 97: pp 705-709

36. *Aromatherapy for Everyone*, Tisserand (Arkana, 1990), pp 113-144, 176-179

37. *Mint Condition*, Griggs (in *Country Living*, August 1991) pp 126-128

38. *Herbs* (Herb Society journal), autumn/winter 1990, pp 10-13

39. Dooms-Goossens et al, *Contact Dermatitis*, 1977; 3: pp 304-308

40. Luke, *Lancet*,1962: pp 110-111

41. O'Mullane et al, *Lancet*, 1982,1/8281: 1121

42. Thomas, *Lancet*, 1962: p 222

43. *Understanding the Irritable Bowel Syndrome* (British Digestive Foundation), p 9

44. Jones and Lydeard, *British Medical Journal*, 1992, 304: pp 87-90

45. Nash et al, *British Journal of Clinical Practice*, 1986; 40: pp 292-293

46. Lawson et al, *Journal of Gastroenterology and Hepatology*, 1988; 3: pp 235-238

47. Lech et al, *Ugeskrift For Laeger*, October 1988

48. Rees et al, *British Medical Journal*, 1979; 2: pp 835-837

49. Dew et al, *British Journal of Clinical Practice*, 1984; 8: pp 45-48

50. Munst et al, *Therapiewoche Schweiz*, 1987; 9: pp 863-868

51. Carling, *Opuscula Medica*, 1989; 34: pp 55-57

52. Leicester and Hunt, *Lancet*, 1982; ii: p 959

53. Duthie, *British Journal of Surgery*, 1981; 68: p 820

54. Somerville et al, *British Journal of Clinical Pharmacology*, 1984; 18: pp 638-640

55. Krag, *Scandinavian Journal of Gastroenterology*, 1985; 20 Suppl. 109: 107-115

56. *Coping Successfully With Your Irritable Bowel*, Nicol (Sheldon Press, 1991)

57. *Out of the Earth*, Mills (Viking 1991), p 103

58. Gilchrest, *Archives of International Medicine*, 1982; 142: pp 101-105

59. *Physical and Biological Properties of Carminatives*, Evans (PhD, University of Wales)

60. *The Herb Book*, Boxer and Back (Peerage Books, 1985)

Other Sources include:

Secret Remedies and What They Contain (British Medical Association, 1909)

Herbal Prescriptions from a Consultant's Case Book, Burns Lingard (1958)

British Species of Mentha, Smith (1799)

Medicinal Plants of the Bible, Duke (Trado-Medic Books, 1983)

Plants of the Bible, Zohary (CUP, 1982)

Braintree Means Business, pamphlet on John Ray

Anglo-Saxon Herbs and Medicine, St Paul's Jarrow Development Trust

The Complete Book of Herbs, Bremness (Dorling Kindersley, 1988)

Potter's New Cyclopaedia, R. C. Wren (C. W. Daniel, 1988)

The Dictionary of Healing Plants, Dorfler and Roselt (Blandford Press, 1989)

Guide to Medicinal Plants, Schauenberg and Paris (Keats Publishing, 1977)

The Home Herbal, Griggs (Hale, 1986)

The Fragrant Pharmacy, Worwood (Bantam, 1991)

L'Aromathérapie Exactement, Franchome, Penoël

Martindales, *The Extra Pharmacopoeia* (Pharmaceutical Press, 1989)

Principles of Anatomy and Physiology, Tortora and Anagnostakos (Harper and Row, 1984)

Introductory Plant Biology, Stern (Wm C. Brown, 1991)

Fisher, *Reactions to Menthol*, Cutis, 1986; pp 17-18

Weston, *Anal burning and peppermint oil*, Postgraduate Medical Journal, 1987; 63: 717

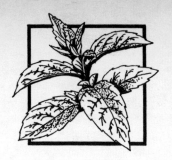

Index